Chikungunya Virus-Like Particles as Vaccine Candidates: A Pilot Study

CHIKUNGUNYA VIRUS-LIKE PARTICLES AS VACCINE CANDIDATES: A PILOT STUDY

Shweta Saraswat and Khushboo Chaudhary

Delve PUBLISHING

www.delvepublishing.com

Chikungunya Virus-Like Particles as Vaccine Candidates: A Pilot Study

Shweta Saraswat and Khushboo Chaudhary

Delve Publishing
224 Shoreacres Road
Burlington, ON L7L 2H2
Canada
www.delvepublishing.com
Email: orders@arclereducation.com

ISBN: 978-1-77469-529-6 (Hardcover)

ABOUT THE AUTHORS

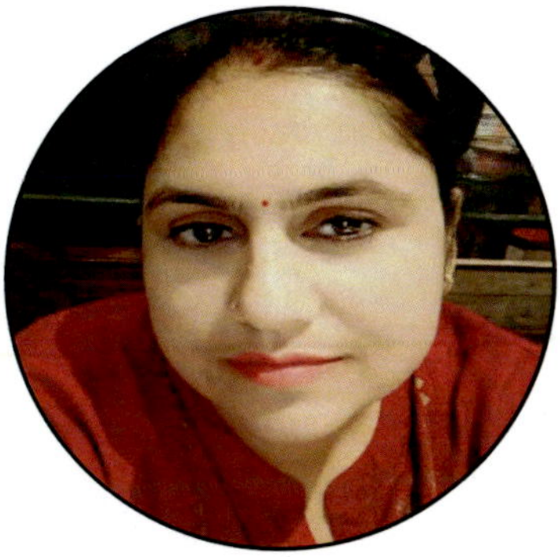

Dr. Shweta Saraswat is currently working as an Assistant Professor at the Amity Institute of Virology and Immunology (AIVI), Amity University, Uttar Pradesh, Noida, India. Dr. Saraswat has 3 years of teaching experience and more than 10 years of research experience. She is a graduate and has a master's in microbiology from Jiwaji University, Gwalior. Dr. Saraswat completed her doctorate in Biological Sciences (Virology) from Bharathiar University, Coimbatore. Her research area was the development of Chikungunya Virus-Like particles using Picha pastoris. She worked in various renowned organizations in India. She worked at the Defence Research and Development Establishment (DRDE), Gwalior as a research fellow. Here, her area of expertise was the development of diagnostics and prophylactics against Chikungunya, Dengue, and Swine flu viruses. She was a postdoctoral fellow at Shiv Nadar University, Gautam Buddha Nagar. Her work was mainly focused on the "Mapping of cleavage site of HEV ORF1 expressed using the Baculovirus expression system". After that, she worked as a scientist at the Translational Health Science and Technology Institute (THSTI), Faridabad, to isolate various DENV isolates using clinical samples. She also identified some small molecule inhibitors against DENV as well as other flaviviruses. At the National Institute of Immunology, her focus was to develop neutralization assays for different JEV isolates. She has been awarded by various reputed agencies. She has received DST-NPDF and DHR-young scientist national awards. She also got an international travel grant from the International Conference on Antiviral Research (ICAR). She also submitted many DENV gene sequences to NCBI Pubmed. Dr. Saraswat has published several research papers in international journals. She is the author and co-author of so many international journals. She is also a review editor for Frontiers in Cellular and Infection Microbiology.

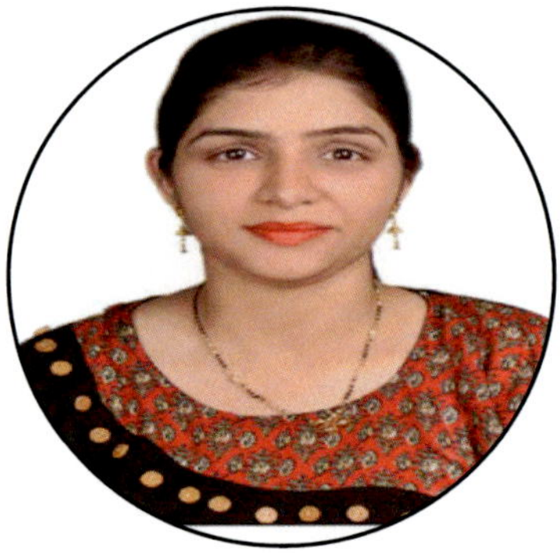

Dr. Khushboo Chaudhary is presently working as a Senior Research Associate at THSTI, Faridabad, Haryana and has nine years of research experience. She graduated from Dr. M.P.S College, Agra in 2010, completed post-graduation from R.B.S College, Agra (Dr. Bhim Rao Ambedkar University) in 2012 and Ph.D. in Biotechnology from Banasthali Vidyapith Tonk Rajasthan in 2019. She has published several research papers in international and national journals. She has published six international textbooks. She has received seven best paper and poster presentation awards from the Indian Society of Genetics and Biotechnology Research and Development and received the president appreciation awards also in the International Conference. She has got the best poster award from ISSGPU Central Institute Research on Goats, Makhdoom. She has published several gene banks in NCBI Pubmed. She has also published a research article in the virology journal. She is likely to be a co-author in several of the publications and coauthor in J. Virological Methods.

TABLE OF CONTENTS

LIST OF ABBREVIATIONS

ANOVA	:	Analysis of Variance
APS	:	Ammonium Persulfate
BCA	:	Bicinchoninic Acid Assay
BLAST	:	Basic Local Alignment Search Tool
β-ME	:	Beta Mercaptoethanol
bp	:	Base pair
BSA	:	Bovine serum albumin
BSL-3	:	Biosafety level-3 containment facility
CO_2	:	Carbon Dioxide
CDC	:	Center for Disease Control and Prevention, Atlanta
Con A	:	Concanavalin A
C-terminal	:	Carboxy terminal
CPE	:	Cytopathic Effect
CHIKV	:	Chikungunya virus
CHIKE2	:	Chikungunya virus envelope protein E2
DAB	:	Diaminobenzidine
DENV	:	Dengue Virus
DMSO	:	Dimethyl Sulfoxide
DNA	:	Deoxyribonucleic Acid
DTT	:	Dithiothreitol
E. coli	:	*Escherichia coli*
EDTA	:	Ethylenediaminetetracetic acid
ELISA	:	Enzyme linked immunosorbent assay
EMEM	:	Eagle's Minimum Essential Medium
EU	:	Endotoxin units
FDA	:	Food and Drug Administration
FCA	:	Freund's complete adjuvant

FIA	:	Freund's incomplete adjuvant
FITC	:	Fluorescein isothiocyanate
H_2O_2	:	Hydrogen peroxide
HIS	:	Hyper immune sera
hpi	:	Hours Post Infection
HRP	:	Horse Radish Peroxidase
IAEC	:	Institutional Animal Ethics Committee
IFN-γ	:	Interferon-γ
IFT	:	Immunofluorescence Test
IgG	:	Immunoglobulin G
IL	:	Interleukin
JEV	:	Japanese Encephalitis virus
kb	:	Kilo base pairs
kDa	:	Kilo Dalton
Kan	:	Kanamycin
LAL	:	Limulus Amoebocyte Lysates
LB	:	Luria bertani broth
LD50	:	Lethal Dose-50
µg	:	Microgram
µl	:	Microliter
µm	:	Micromolar
mg	:	Milligram
MAb	:	Monoclonal antibody
M.O.I	:	Multiplicity of Infection
mRNA	:	Messenger RNA
N-terminal	:	Amino terminal
ng	:	Nanogram
NFW	:	Nuclease Free Water
NS	:	Non-structural Protein
O.D.	:	Optical Density
PAGE	:	Polyacrylamide Gel Electrophoresis
PAb	:	Polyclonal antibody
PBS	:	Phosphate Buffered Saline
PBST	:	Phosphate Buffered Saline with Tween-20

PMSF	:	Phenylmethyl sulfonyl fluoride
P. pastoris:		*Pichia pastoris*
PRNT	:	Plaque reduction neutralization test
Pfu	:	*Pyrococcus furiosus*
PFU	:	Plaque forming unit
qPCR	:	Quantitative Real Time PCR
RNA	:	Ribose Nucleic Acid
Rpm	:	Rotations per Minute
RT	:	Room temperature
RT-PCR	:	Reverse Transcriptase Polymerase Chain Reaction
SAv-HRP:		Streptavidin–horseradish peroxidase conjugate
SD	:	Standard Deviation
SDS	:	Sodium Dodecyl Sulphate
SDS- PAGE:		Sodium Dodecyl Sulphate Polyacrylamide GelElectrophoresis
ssRNA	:	Single-Stranded Ribonucleic Acid
Taq	:	*Thermus aquaticus*
Tm	:	Melting Temperature
TEMED	:	N, N, N', N'-Tetramethylethylenediamine
TMB	:	3,3',5,5'-tetramethylbenzidine
TNF-α	:	Tumor-necrosis factor-α
UV	:	Ultraviolet
Vero	:	African green monkey kidney cell line
VLPs	:	Virus-Like Particles
vRNP	:	Viral Ribonucleoprotein
WHO	:	World Health Organization

PREFACE

The book "**Chikungunya Virus-Like Virus-Like Particles**" has been written to serve as a textbook for postgraduate and research scholars from different universities. The introduction to the Chikungunya virus and its scopes are covered in the first chapter. The second chapter discusses the classification and transmission cycle of the virus and the third chapter explains how to construct particles that resemble the Chikungunya virus. This was confirmed using molecular-based technology, which is described in the fourth chapter. A summary of the chikungunya virus-like particles is presented in the fifth chapter. This book contains a tremendous amount of virus-related experimental material.

All the chapters on Chikungunya Virus-Like particles have been amended, as well as several experiments are described. The main emphasis continues to be the Chikungunya virus for virology interests, although they have been described in specific cases where more is known about the mechanism of Chikungunya virus replication. The chapters have been organized in such a way that they provide sequential knowledge. The names of scientists and authors have been quoted or fully acknowledged and referenced at the end of the book. Shweta Saraswat confirms study conceptualization, validation and design of the manuscript and Khushboo Chaudhary reviewed and edited the final version of this book manuscript. In the preparation of this book, I have been greatly helped by several books and publications, which I have acknowledged in the references. If I have forgotten any references in my notice, please forgive the same. Comments and suggestions are most welcome.

Shweta Saraswat

Khushboo Chaudhary

CHAPTER 1

INTRODUCTION AND SCOPE OF CHIKUNGUNYA VIRUS-LIKE PARTICLES

INTRODUCTION

Chikungunya virus (CHIKV) has now emerged as one of the most important arbovirus of public health significance. Infection of CHIKV in humans is characterized by rash, high fever and severe arthritis that may persist for years. A novel strain of CHIKV appeared in Kenya in 2005 and has spread in many parts of Asia, Africa and Europe. Recently it was also reported from Caribbean islands and Americas (Alessandra et al., 2014).

CHIKV is an enveloped virus and its genome consists of a positive-sense, single- stranded RNA molecule of approximately 12kb encoding two open reading frames (ORF). The ORF located at the 5'end of the genome encodes a polyprotein precursor of nonstructural proteins (nsP1, nsP2, nsP3, nsP4) with replicative and proteolytic activities. The second ORF encodes the polyprotein precursor of the structural proteins (C, E1, E2) involved in viral capsid assembly (Strauss & Strass, 1994). Phylogenetically CHIKV has been classified into three genotypes: Asian, East-Central-South-African and West African. CHIKV is transmitted mainly by *Aedes aegypti* and *Ae. albopictus* mosquitoes. The vector control measures that can play important role in the control of infection is proved unsuccessful in many parts of the world (Stephen & Dana, 2015). Currently, there are no licensed antiviral or vaccines available commercially. There is also a scarcity of reliable diagnostic kits in endemic areas, making disease management and virus transmission check extremely difficult.

The routine laboratory diagnosis of CHIKV infection is based on virus isolation, molecular assays (RT-PCR) and serology. Both virus isolation and RT-PCR though highly specific, are technically demanding and currently restricted to referral laboratories. Serologically, CHIKV diagnosis relies on the detection of IgM and IgG antibodies through ELISA and immunochromatography test (ICT). In view of large-scale epidemic potential of CHIKV, there is a need to develop fast high throughput serological diagnostic assays which are amenable to remote settings. The success of serological assays inherently depends on the quality of the antigen. Replacement of cell culture-derived native CHIKV antigen by recombinant virus protein leads to improved specificity, however, the limitation includes compromised sensitivity, due to the availability of limited immunogenic epitopes (Sam et al., 2015).

The Virus-Like particles (VLPs) are non-infectious, nanosized caged structures composed of viral structural proteins (Roldao et al., 2010; Schwarz et al., 2015). The presence of complete structural proteins makes it an excellent antigen that strongly mimics the native virus. Currently available commercial ELISA and ICT kits suffer from the issues of poor sensitivity and specificity and many products were withdrawn from the market (Prat et al., 2014). The VLPs-based diagnostic assay provides a promising alternative for the detection of CHIKV infection with a high degree of sensitivity and specificity (Schwarz et al., 2015).

The first CHIKV vaccine prototype was a formalin-inactivated virus and later live-attenuated virus vaccines have also been developed in the early 1980s. Though live- attenuated vaccines have the advantage of inducing an efficient, balanced immune response, they have a risk of reversion to virulence (Noad and Roy, 2003). Current research initiatives following the reemergence of CHIKV has led to the development of chimeric vaccines, DNA vaccines, adenoviral vectored vaccines and subunit protein vaccine candidates. However, these candidates have their own complications in manufacturing, immunogenicity, safety, recombination and large-scale production (Kutzler et al., 2008). None of these vaccines are yet successfully completed clinical trials. Recent studies have shown promising results in the development of a CHIK-VLPs-based vaccine that elicited adequate neutralizing antibody response (Akhata et al., 2010; Metz et al., 2013; Ahola et al., 2015). The role of neutralizing antibodies in the protection against CHIKV infection is already well documented (Weaver et al., 2012).

The production platform of choice for the expression of recombinant protein should be safe to use, reach high production yields and be industrially scalable. Prokaryotic systems are not suitable for the expression of viral protein due to the absence of post- translational modification (Bryne, 2015). Yeast represents an alternate eukaryotic expression system for the generation of virus glycoproteins. Yeast as an expression host offers distinct advantages over mammalian and insect expression systems both in terms of scalability and productivity as well as the proven safety of yeast-derived viral proteins free from viral contamination for pharmaceutical applications, e.g. hepatitis B vaccine (Cregg et al., 2000). In this study, the methylotrophic yeast *Pichia pastoris* was selected to express Chikungunya virus structural proteins. *P. pastoris* has been used to express a number of therapeutic proteins that have even entered clinical trials (Gerngross et al., 2004; Bryne, 2015).

SCOPE OF CHIK-VLPS

The continuous expansion of CHIKV and increase in human morbidity make it one of the most important emerging arboviruses. There is a demand to develop a safe and economical diagnostic assay for screening of a large number of patients during the time of epidemics. Further, a safe and effective CHIKV vaccine is clearly needed to protect humans and also to stop CHIKV transmission. Several strategies have been designed to combat CHIKV infections but none of these have been licensed yet and are not easily amenable to scale up. The purpose of this study is to design and develop a novel CHIKV immunogen that can be employed for both diagnostic and prophylactic applications. Quality of antigen plays the most crucial role in the development of a diagnostic system. VLPs owing to their close conformational resemblance to the native virus provide the best quality of antigen further obviating biosafety concerns. It has also shown the ability to induce both humoral and cell-mediated immune responses. Yeast (*Pichia pastoris*) based expression system is now widely adopted for the expression of viral proteins intended for both diagnostic and prophylactic applications.

Keeping in view these facts, the present study was undertaken to develop an advanced VLPs -based new generation diagnostic and vaccine candidate with the following objectives:

- A two-step purification strategy for Chikungunya virion using sucrose buoyant density gradient separation
- Heterologous expression and characterization of CHIK-VLPs using *Pichia pastoris.*

- Evaluation of CHIK-VLPs as a diagnostic intermediate in serological diagnosis.

Evaluation of the immunogenic potential of CHIK-VLPs in BALB/c mice.

CHAPTER 2

OVERVIEW OF CHIKUNGUNYA VIRUS

INTRODUCTION

Arbovirus and Its Emergence

Arthropod-borne viruses (arboviruses) are important causes of human disease nearly worldwide. These are transmitted biologically among vertebrate hosts by hematophagous (blood feeding) arthropod vectors such as mosquitoes and other biting flies, and ticks. Being, by definition, biologically transmitted, arboviruses must replicate in the arthropod vector prior to transmission, as opposed to being mechanically transmitted, without replication in the vector, through contaminated mouthparts (Weaver, 1997).

The arboviruses include a wide variety of RNA virus taxa including the *alphaviruses,* the *Flaviviruses*, *Bunyaviruses, Nairoviruses*, *Phleboviruses*, *Orbiviruses*, *Vesiculoviruses* and *Thogotoviruses. Arboviruses* circulate among wild animals, and cause disease after spillover transmission to humans and/or domestic animals that are incidental or dead-end hosts. Viruses such as dengue (DENV) and chikungunya (CHIKV) that have lost the requirement for enzootic amplification now produce extensive epidemics.

Many *Arboviruses* that have evolved and diversified in the tropics have produced virulent and invasive strains that have caused major outbreaks at temperate latitudes. All *Arboviruses* circulate among wild animals, and many cause disease after spillover transmission to humans and agriculturally important domestic animals that are incidental or dead-end hosts. Viruses such as dengue (DENV) and chikungunya (CHIKV) viruses that have lost the requirement for enzootic amplification now produce extensive epidemics in tropical urban centers. Many arboviruses recently have increased in importance as human and veterinary pathogens using a variety of mechanisms (Weaver et al., 2010).

Classification of Chikungunya Virus

Chikungunya virus (CHIKV) is an alphavirus that belongs to family *Togaviridae.* About 30 species of arthropod-borne viruses are included in the alphavirus genus, antigenically classified into 7 complexes. These viruses are widely distributed throughout the world, with the exception of Antarctica. CHIKV is a member of the Semliki Forest Virus (SFV) complex and is closely related to Ross River Virus, Mayaro, O' Nyong Nyong virus, Getha, Bebru and Semliki Forest Virus. In the United States, it is classified as a Category C priority pathogen and work requires biosafety level 3 precautions (Taubiz et al., 2007).

CHIKV Structure

CHIKV is a small (about 60–70 nm-diameter), spherical, enveloped, positive- strand RNA virus. The RNA is encapsidated in a ~40 nm wide nucleocapsid, which is enveloped by a host-derived lipid bilayer supporting 80 viral trimeric glycoprotein-spikes, which are involved in cell receptor recognition and cell entry via low pH-dependent fusion and endocytosis (Strauss & Strauss, 1994; Powers et al., 2001; Khan et al. 2002).

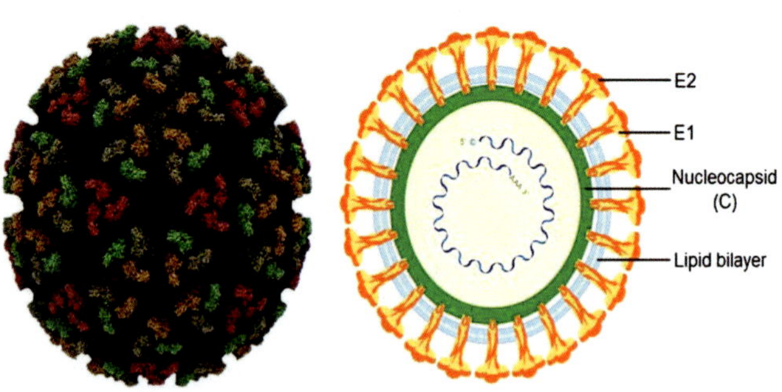

Figure 2.1: CHIKV virion (generated from Protein Data Bank data, based on Sindbis EM density, PDB ID: 2XFB) and schematic representation of CHIKV particle section. Reproduced from Metz and Pijlman, 2011.

CHIKV Genome

The genome of CHIKV is organized as: 5′ cap-nsP1-nsP2-nsP3-nsP4-(junction region)-C-E3-E2-6k-E1-poly(A)-3′ and is 11,805 nucleotides long, excluding the 5′ cap nucleotide, an I-poly(A) tract and the 3′ poly(A) tail. It contains two open reading frames (ORF) encoding the non-structural polyprotein and the structural polyprotein. The non- structural proteins (nsP1-4) regulate viral RNA replication and are directly translated from the 5'end of the genome. The structural proteins (Capsid or C, envelope proteins E3, E2, 6K, E1) constitute the virion proteins and are translated from a subgenomic mRNA located in the 3'-end of the genome (Strauss & Strauss, 1994).

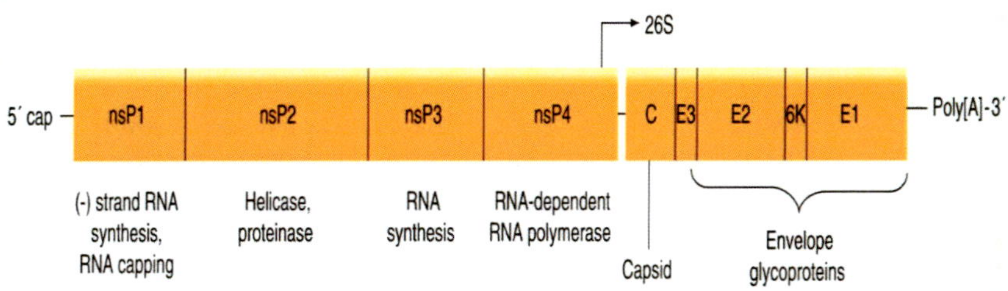

Figure 2.2: Genomic organization of the CHIKV. The four non-structural proteins (nsP1– 4) are translated as a single polyprotein directly from the positive-sense RNA genome. The structural proteins (C, E3, E2, 6K and E1) are translated from a subgenomic RNA (26S) transcribed from a separate promoter within the non-translated (NTR) junction region. 5' and 3' NTR region flanks the coding region. Reproduced from Weaver et al., 2012.

The genomic RNA acts as cellular messenger RNA. Therefore, the 5' end is capped with a 7-methylguanosine, while the 3' end is polyadenylated. The 5′-non- translatable regions (NTR) of CHIKV are composed of 76 nucleotides while the 3′-NTR of CHIKV is composed of 526 nucleotides.

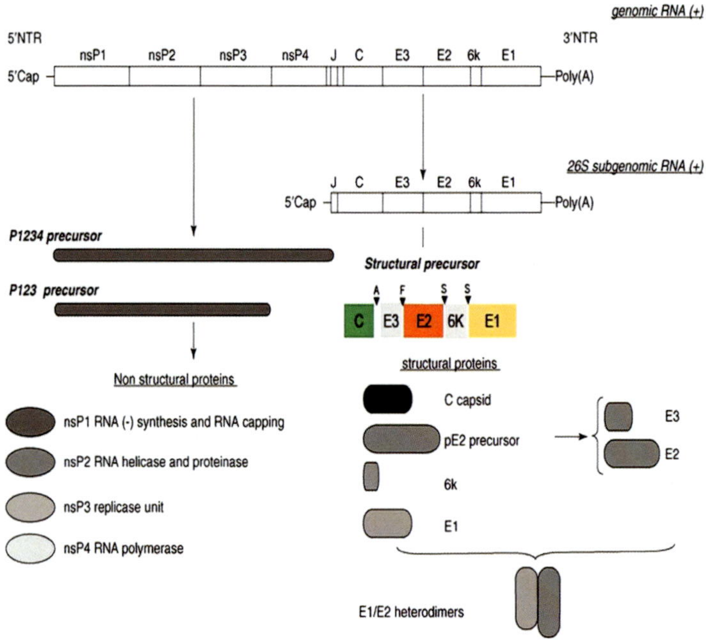

Figure 2.3: CHIKV genome and its products. Reproduced from Chevillon et al., 2007.

The nonstructural domain of 7425 nt, covering the first two-thirds of the genomic RNA, which are directly translated into the non-structural proteins and a structural domain of 3732 nt covering the last third of the genome, encoding the structural proteins of the virus. Both the open reading frame (ORF) can be cleaved respectively into four non-structural proteins (nsP1, nsP2, nsP3, nsP4) and five structural proteins (C, E3, E2, 6K, E1) by viral and cellular proteases (Khan et al., 2002).

Non-structural Proteins

It includes nsP1, nsP2, nsP3 and nsP4 proteins. The nonstructural proteins are required for the transcription and replication of the viral RNA. In the early stage of infection, the non-structural proteins are synthesized directly from two-thirds of genomic RNA as a P1234 polypeptide and in the process of replication, this polyprotein is cleaved to form all four nonstructural proteins: nsP1, nsP2, nsP3 and nsP4. These all proteins play different roles in the life cycle of CHIKV.

nsP1 - It is 535 amino acids long. nsP1 is involved in the synthesis of the negative strand of viral RNA and has RNA capping properties and also to be involved in the association of the replication complex to cellular membranes (Griffin et al., 1997).

nsP2- nsP2 displays RNA helicase, RNA trisphosphatase and proteinase activities and cleaves the non-structural polyprotein to form the individual non-structural proteins (Strauss et al., 1992) and are also involved in the shut-off of host cell transcription (Garmashova et al., 2007).

nsP3 - It is 530 amino acids long. The function of nsP3 in viral replication remains largely unknown. It is part of the replicase unit and essential for minus-strand and subgenomic 26S mRNA synthesis (Strauss et al., 1994).

nsP4 -611 amino acid long protein and is the viral RNA polymerase and interacts with the N-terminal region and other non-structural proteins and unknown host cellular factors (Griffin et al., 2007).

Structural Proteins

The structural proteins, capsid, E3, E2, 6K and E1, are synthesized from a sub- genomic mRNA as a single polypeptide, which is cleaved both co-translationally and post-translationally to form structural proteins (Strauss et al., 1986; Faragher et al., 1988; Strauss et al., 1988). These structural proteins have important functions in the replication of the virus and particularly in the interaction with the host. This interaction resulted in the production of antibodies which played important roles in the recovery from infection (Griffin et al., 1997). Antibodies can neutralize virus infectivity and reduce the viral load by the complement systems (Jahrling et al., 1983). The junction region is located in between the nonstructural and structural domains and functions to promote transcription of an intracellular subgenomic 26S RNA. In addition to the junction region, there are two other untranslated regions: one at the 5'-end, which is required for plus-strand RNA synthesis (Strauss et al., 1994) and the other which is located at the 3' end between the stop codon of the E1 gene and the poly (A) tail. This region is mainly involved in the translation of viral proteins rather than in the replication of the genomic RNA (Leathers et al., 1993).

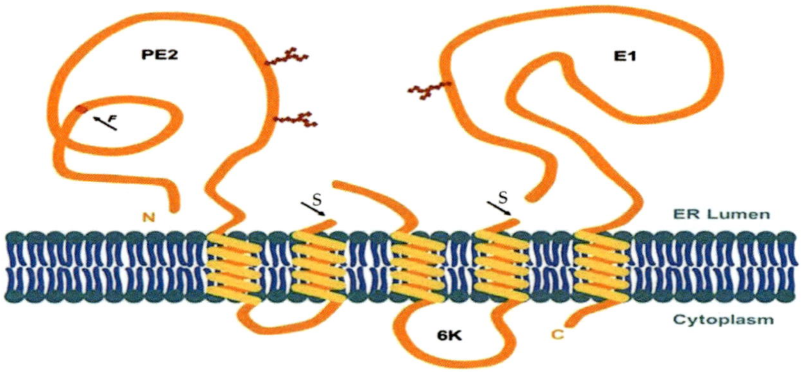

Figure 2.4: CHIKV trimeric spike structure. A) Schematic representation of ER- membrane organization of the CHIKV envelope cassette. N- and C-terminal ends are indicated. Arrows represent cleavage sites for S (host signalases) and F (furin-like proteases). Blue chains indicate N-glycosylation sites (Metz and Pijlman, 2011).

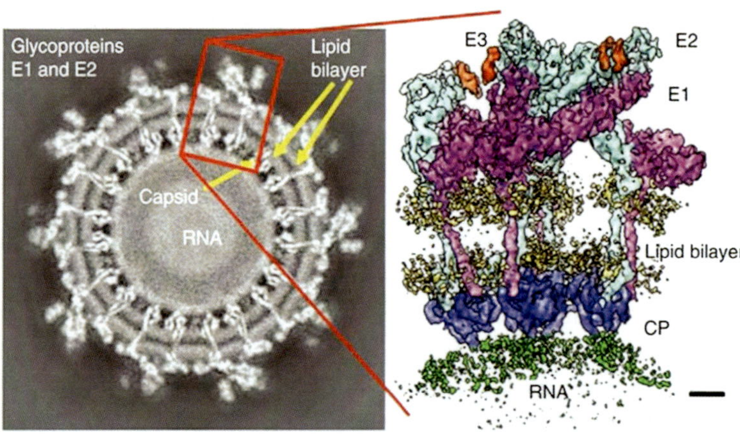

Figure 2.5: Chikungunya virus showing the orientation of E1, E2, E3 and Capsid protein. Cryo-EM density of an alphavirus trimeric spike, with E3 (orange) incorporated in the spike composed of E2 (cyan), E1 (magenta) and capsid (blue). Viral RNA (green) and the host-derived lipid bilayer (yellow) are also depicted (Zhang et al., 2011).

E1- The E1 protein contained 435 amino acids and has a molecular weight of 44 kDa. Contains one glycosylation site at position 141, It is a class II viral fusion protein (Zhang et al., 2011; Cho et al., 2008b).

E2 –It contains 423 amino acids and has a molecular weight of 43 kDa. The E2 protein had two possible glycosylation sites at positions 263 and 345 assigned by the sequence Asn-X-Ser/Thr (where X is any amino acid except proline). It is responsible for viral attachment to the target host cell, by binding to the cell receptor (Zhang et al., 2011; Cho et al., 2008b).

E3 –It is a small protein having 64 amino acids and its function has not been studied so far, yet it could share disulfide isomerase activity recently described for SINV E3 protein that could be involved in proper folding and disulfide bound formation in viral envelope glycoprotein spike formation (Parrott et al., 2009). E3 of CHIKV is not associated with virions but is released from infected cells (Simizuet al., 1984).

Capsid –The capsid protein of CHIKV is 261 amino acids long and has a molecular weight of 30 kDa. It possesses protease activity that results in its autocatalytic cleavage from the nascent structural protein (Cho et al., 2008a).

6K protein- It is postulated to influence the selection of lipids that interact with the transmembrane domains of the glycoproteins, which, in turn, affects the deformability of the bilayer required for the extreme curvature that occurs as budding proceeds (Simizu et al., 1984).

Replication Cycle

Chikungunya virus enters host cells by clathrin-dependent endocytosis (Griffin 2007) but the receptors are still not known. Rab5 plays an important role in this transport the function of which is mainly to recycle receptors and is required for the transport of the early endosome along the microtubule. Following endocytosis, the acidic environment of the endosome triggers conformational changes in the viral envelope that expose the E1 protein surface (Kielian & Helenius, 2006) which mediates virus–host cell membrane fusion. This allows the release of the viral genome (Powers et al., 2001) and core in the host cell cytoplasm. In CHIKV, the initial translation of the non-structural region generates two polyproteins P123 and P1234. P1234 is produced due to a read-through strategy (due to a leaky stop signal) at the C-terminus of nsp3 (Ding and Schlesinger, 1989). *In cis*- cleavage of P1234, yields P123 and nsP4, the viral RNA-dependent RNA-polymerase (RdRp). After or in parallel to the emergence of nsP4, nsP1 is presumably cleaved off from P123, yielding nsP1, P23 and nsP4. The nsp4 functions as a polymerase for both plus- and minus-strand RNA, but minus-strand RNA is only generated in the presence of P123. Thus nsP1, P23 and nsP4 act together as the minus-strand RNA replication complex. After further processing of P23 into nsP2 and nsP3 in trans-cleavage by nsP2, the template preference of the replicase is altered to minus-stranded RNA, thereby promoting the synthesis of plus-strand and subgenomic RNA. This shut-off mechanism of minus-strand RNA synthesis is tightly regulated by nsP2 since no viral RNA replication is observed with increased P123 processing efficiency and minus-stranded RNA accumulates with inactivated nsP2 (Lemm et al., 1994).

During the translation of the structural polyprotein from a subgenomic viral mRNA, C is autocatalytically cleaved off and the remaining envelope cassette is translocated to the ER by signal sequences in E3 and 6K. Proteolytic processing by host signalases cleaves 6K at the N-and C-terminal end, yielding E3E2 (precursor E2 or PE2), 6K and E1 (Kuhn, 2007). Following processing, PE2 and E1 form heterodimers, which are assembled into heterotrimers in the early Golgi compartment. Subsequently, E3 is released from PE2 by furin-dependent cleavage and maturation in the trans-Golgi system receiving glycosylation. Furin cleavage is not a prerequisite for virion assembly, but incomplete processing will result in virions with impaired fusion properties (Strauss et al., 1994). The mature heterotrimers are displayed at the cell-surface as trimeric spikes and the viral RNA is encapsidated in nucleocapsids composed of 240 copies of C (Weiss et al., 1989).

Virion budding is most likely regulated by the interaction between the intracellular domain of E2 with a single C molecule within the nucleocapsid (Garoff et al., 2004). The nucleocapsid buds out from the cell, taking along the hosts' plasma membrane and a total of 80 trimeric spikes (Garoff et al., 2004). The trimeric spikes are essential for cell-receptor recognition (E2) and pH-dependent endocytosis (E1). Upon receptor binding, conformational changes in E2 trigger the onset of E1 homotrimer formation, after which the mild acidic conditions in the endosome induce membrane fusion (Gibbons et al., 2000).

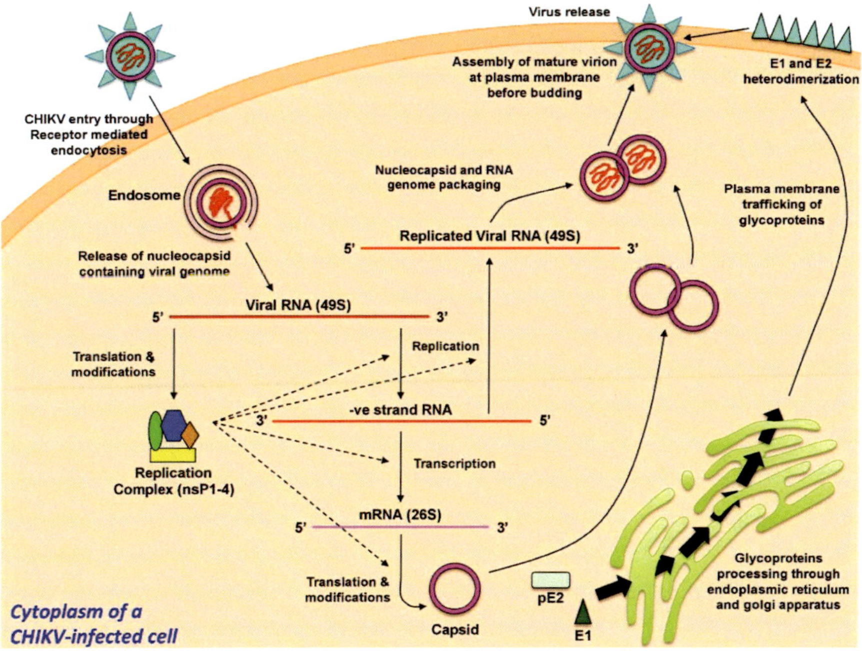

Figure 2.6: CHIKV replication cycle (Lum & Ng, 2015).

The virus enters susceptible cells through endocytosis, mediated by an unknown receptor. As the endosome is acidic, conformational changes occur resulting in the fusion of the viral and host cell membranes, causing the release of the nucleocapsid into the cytoplasm, The RNA genome is first translated into the 4 nsPs, which together will form the replication complex and assist in several downstream processes (depicted by dashed arrowed line). Subsequently, the genome is replicated to its negative-sense strand, which in turn will be used as a template for the synthesis of the 49S viral RNA and 26S subgenomic mRNA. The 26S subgenomic mRNA will be translated to give the structural proteins (C–E2–6K–E1). After a round of processing by serine proteases, the capsid is released into the cytoplasm. The remaining structural proteins are further modified post- translationally in the endoplasmic reticulum and subsequently in the Golgi apparatus. E1 and E2 associate as a dimer and are transported to the host plasma membrane, where they will ultimately be incorporated onto the virion surface as trimeric spikes. Capsid protein will form the icosahedral nucleocapsid that will contain the replicated 49S genomic RNA before being assembled into a mature virion ready for budding. During budding the virions will acquire a membrane bilayer from part of the host cell membrane (Lum et.al., 2015).

It would be detrimental for the virus if E1 assembles into homotrimers before the trimeric spikes have reached the cell surface. To prevent this from happening, PE2 acts as a chaperone and initially forms heterodimers with the downstream encoded E1. This enables transport to the Golgi apparatus and delaying or preventing premature E1 self- aggregation (Andersson et al., 1997). E2 is not able to form dimers with E1 in the absence of E3. Then E1 is retained in the ER and no further processing will take place. Presumably, PE2 protects the immature trimeric spike from undergoing conformational changes in the acidic Golgi environment, due to interactions between E3 and the top domain of E1 (Lobigs et al., 1990). E3 is not cleaved from PE2, due to inefficient furin processing, E1 can only exert its fusogenic activity at a pH < 5.0, which is lower than the normal intracellular pH-range of= 5.5-5.8. Sporadically, E3 remains associated with the trimeric spike after efficient furin processing of pE2. This, however, will not impede E1 from forming homotrimers (Wu et al., 2008).

Vectors and Reservoir

Chikungunya virus is transmitted by culicinae mosquitoes and can alternatively affect vertebrates and arthropods (Barrett, 2002; Brooks, 2004). The arthropod remains infected throughout all its life. Its transmission to humans is mainly through *Aedes* species of mosquitoes although *Culex* has also been reported for the transmission in rare cases (Diallo et al., 1999; Vanlandingham et al.. 2005; Schuffenecker et al., 2006). In Asia and the Indian Ocean region, the main CHIKV vectors are *Aedes aegypti* and *Aedes albopictus* (Zeller, 1998; Jeandel et al., 2004). A larger range of *Aedes* species (*A. furcifer, A. vittatus, A. fulgens, A. luteocephalus, A. dalzieli, A. vigilax, A. camptorhynchites, A. polynesiensis*) transmit the virus in Africa, and *Culex annulirostris, Mansonia uniformis,* and *Anopheles* mosquitoes have also occasionally been incriminated (Jupp & McIntosh, 1990; Lam et al., 2001). The common reservoirs for the Chikungunya virus are monkeys and other vertebrates. The role of cattle and rodents has also been reported in the transmission of CHIKV (Alessandra et al., 2014; Diallo et al., 1999).

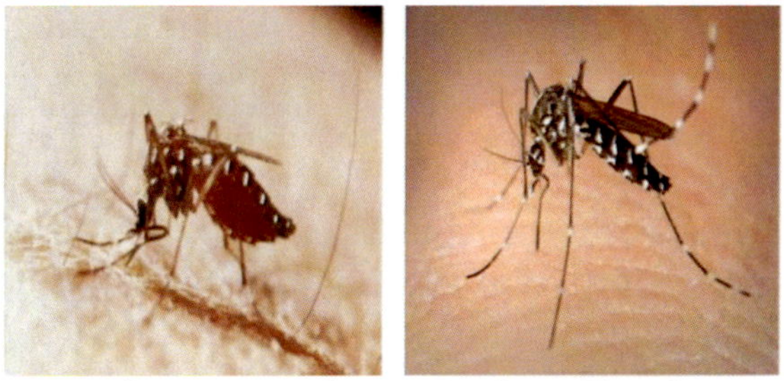

Aedes aegypti ***Aedes albopictus***

Figure 2.7: Vectors of Chikungunya virus. These mosquitoes can be identified by the white stripes on their black bodies and legs. A female *Ae. aegypti* (right) and a female *Ae. albopictus* (left) feeding on a human (Image Centers for Disease Control Public Health Image Library).

In India, the dominant carrier of the Chikungunya virus is *A. aegypti*, which breeds mainly in stored fresh water in urban and semi-urban environments. It seems that most new introductions of *A. albopictus* have been caused by vegetative eggs contained in timber and tyres exported from Asia throughout the world. The *A. albopictus* population is very high, particularly in southern coastal states and it has played an important role in the transmission of mutant CHIKV in India (Caglioti et al., 2013).

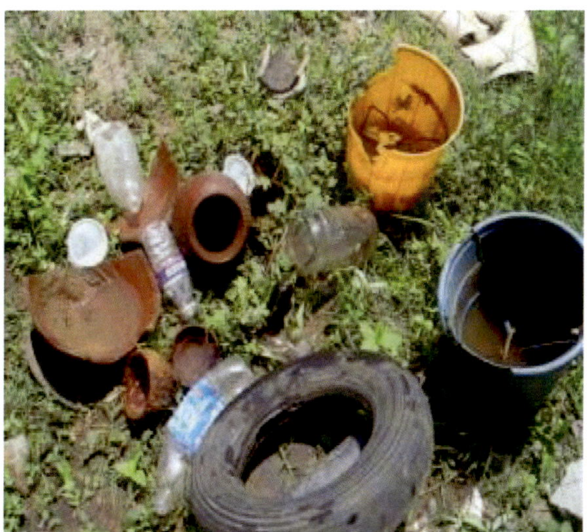

Figure 2.8: Reservoir of CHIKV vector: The mosquito mainly breeds on stored fresh water in tyres, buckets, flower pots and bottles. Reproduced from http://health.puducherry.gov.in/FAQ/Chikungunya.htm

Other emerging events also contributed to the introduction of *A. albopictus* mosquitoes into previously unaffected areas, such as climate change and the increasing use of plastic containers in developing countries. Indeed, climate changes may have several effects on vector biology: increasing temperatures may improve survival at higher latitudes and altitudes, increase the growth rates of vector populations, and alter their seasonality; increased rainfall may have an effect on the larval habitat and population size, and finally, an increase in humidity could favorably affect vector survival (Gubler et al., 2001).

Transmission Cycle

There are two epidemiological transmission cycles of CHIKV:

- An enzootic sylvatic cycle
- An endemic/epidemic urban cycle.

The sylvatic cycle occurs primarily in West and South Africa involving mainly wild non-human primates as reservoirs or amplifying hosts and forest dwelling arboreal *Aedes* mosquitoes as a vector where humans are accidental hosts. The major species involved in sylvatic cycles are *A. furcifer, A. vittatus, A. fulgens, A. luteocephalus, A. dalzieli, A. vigilax,* and *A. camptorhynchites*. In Africa, the enzootic transmission cycle can spill over to infect people who live nearby, and enzootic mosquito vectors may be involved in inter- human transmission during small outbreaks. *A. furcifer*, probably a principal enzootic vector, is known to enter human villages (Diallo et al., 1999), where it presumably transmits the virus from monkeys to humans (Peyrefitte et al., 2007; Peyrefitte et al., 2008). This transmission cycle generally results in smaller-scale outbreaks.

An urban human-mosquito-human transmission cycle typically occurs in cities in Asia. The urban transmission cycle relies only on *A. aegypti* and/or *A. albopictus,* anthropophilic vectors that can initiate and sustain human-mosquito-human transmission, and human amplification hosts. This endemic/ epidemic cycle results in high levels of human exposure to mosquito transmission, particularly because these vectors live in close proximity to people. The behavior and ecology of *A. aegypti,* in particular, are ideal for epidemic transmission because adult females prefer to feed on humans, often take several blood meals during a single gonotrophic cycle, oviposit in artificial containers as their preferred larval sites, and rest inside houses with ready access to human hosts (Weaver et al., 2012).

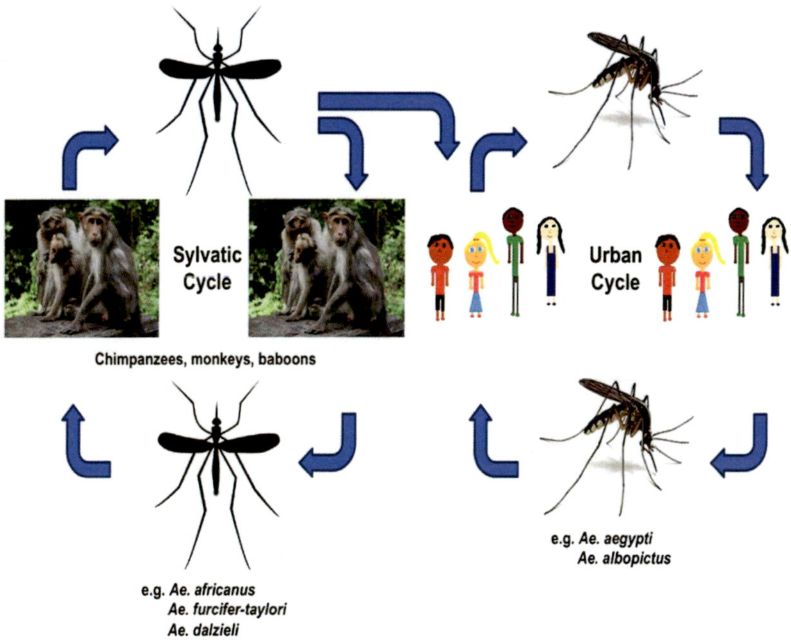

Figure 2.9: Life cycle of Chikungunya virus in Africa showing the interconnection between the sylvatic cycle on the left and the urban cycle on the right (Diallo et al., 1999).

Virus Dissemination and Target Organs in Vertebrate Host

Following intradermal inoculation by infected mosquitoes, CHIKV directly enters the subcutaneous capillaries where its replication starts immediately with some viruses infecting susceptible cells in the skin, such as macrophages or fibroblasts and endothelial cells. Local viral replication seems to be minor and limited in time, with the locally produced virus probably being transported to secondary lymphoid organs close to the site of inoculation, where infected migratory cells produce new viruses which can, in turn, infect susceptible resident cells. Even if the host is mounting a response to control the virus in the skin dermis, the virus disseminates quite rapidly in the draining lymph nodes are released into the lymph circulation and then to the blood through the thoracic duct. Once in the blood, the virus will have access to various parts of the body, including the liver, muscle, joints and brain. In these tissues, the infection is associated with marked infiltration of mononuclear cells, including macrophages, which can be considered Trojan horses for virus spread to sanctuary body sites. The pathological events associated with tissue infection are mostly subclinical in the liver (hepatocyte apoptosis) and lymphoid organs (adenopathy), whereas mononuclear cell infiltration and viral replication in the muscles and joints are associated with very strong pain, with some patients presenting arthritis (Dupuis- Maguiraga et al., 2012; Ong et al., 2014).

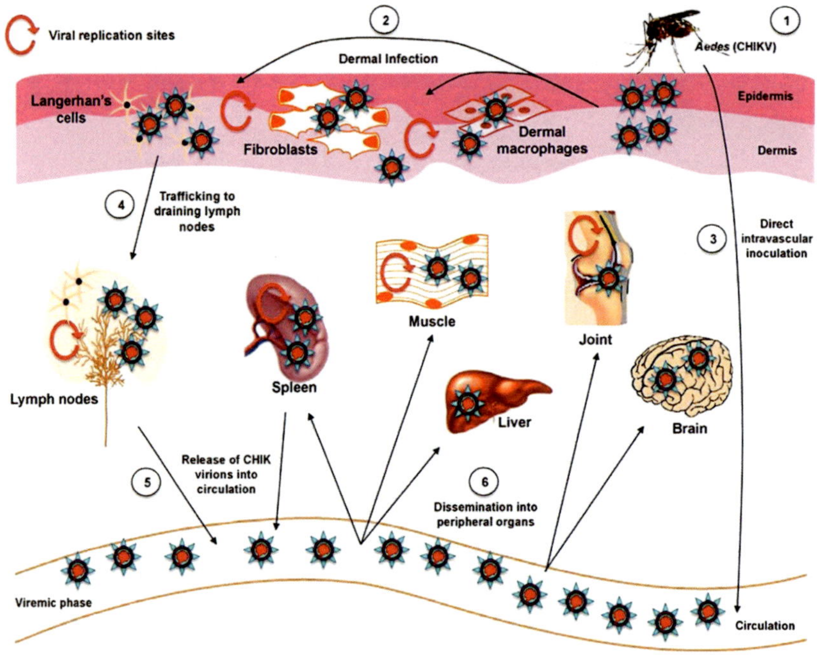

Figure 2.10: Schematic representation of CHIKV dissemination to different tissues and organs. Pathogenesis of CHIKV infection: viral dissemination and impact on host immune response. (1) CHIKV infection occurs through the bite of an infected mosquito, resulting in a (2) dermal infection phase. Skin resident cells become infected, allowing for the initial rounds of replication. (3) Direct inoculation of the virus into the circulation can also occur via mosquito bites. (4) Subsequently, the virus disseminates to draining lymph nodes, where it further replicates before being (5) released into the circulation. (6) It then disseminates to peripheral organs, such as the spleen and muscles, where further replication takes place. permission. Reproduced from Ong et al., 2014.

CHIKV Epidemiology

Global Scenario

CHIKV was first isolated in 1953 during an outbreak in the Newala district of Tanzania. Since the Tanzania outbreak chikungunya virus has caused outbreaks in East Africa (Tanzania and Uganda), Austral Africa (Zimbabwe and East Africa), West Africa (Senegal) and Central Africa (the Central Africa Republic and the Democratic Republic of the Congo). In South East Asia, frequent outbreaks were reported from the 1960s to 2003 in India, Malaysia, Indonesia, Cambodia, Vietnam, Myanmar, Pakistan and Thailand (Chastel, 1963; Jadhav et al., 1965; Nimmannitya et al., 1969; Thaung et al., 1975; Marchette et al., 1978; Thein et al., 1992; Thaikruea et al., 1997; Mourya et al., 2001; Kit, 2002; Laras et al., 2005). Numerous large cities in South East Asia including Calcutta and Bangkok have been identified as particularly active sites of transmission and disease (Pavri, 1964; Sarkar et al., 1965; Burke et al., 1985).

In the later part of the last century, CHIKV outbreaks resurged with major disease clusters documented in Senegal in 1986 and 1996/ 1997, Ivory Coast in 1996/ 1997, DRC during 1998–2000 (Nur et al., 1999; Pastorino et al., 2004), Indonesia in 2003 (Laras et al., 2005), Kenya in 2004, Comoros in 2005, the Seychelles, Mauritius, Madagascar and Re´union islands during 2005–2006 and in India 2006/2007 (Ravi, 2006; Saxena et al., 2006). Outbreaks occurred almost continuously during 2004–2007 with hundreds to thousands of reported cases and new geographical areas involved. Recently, the virus has also crossed the tropics and its presence has been recorded for the first time in the Emilia Romangna Region of northeastern Italy and where the *Aedes albopictus* was implicated as the mosquito vector (Rezza et al., 2007). Cases were reported in Europe (UK, Belgium, Germany, Czech Republic, Norway, Italy, Spain and France), Hong Kong, Canada, Taiwan, Sri Lanka and the USA. These cases were directly associated with the return of tourists from India and affected islands of the Indian Ocean.

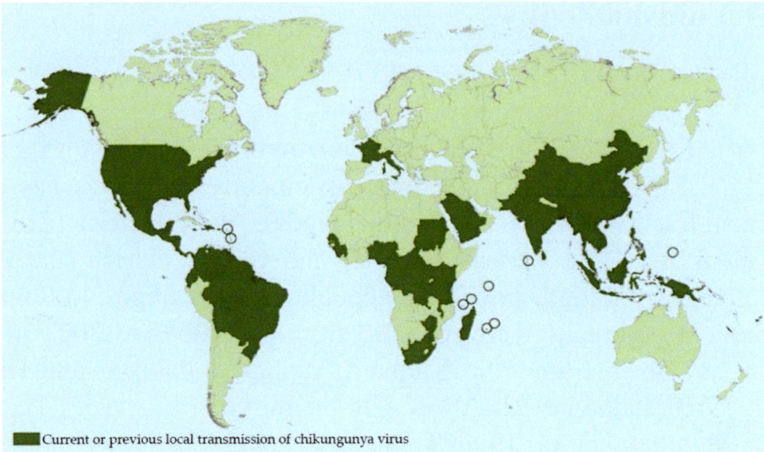

Figure 2.11: Geographic distribution of CHIKV shown in the most recent map (March, 2015) Countries and territories where chikungunya cases have been reported* retrieved from the CDC website (http://www.cdc.gov/chikungunya/map/index.html, last accessed March 2015). *Does not include countries or territories where only imported cases have been documented. This map is updated weekly if there are new countries or territories that report local chikungunya virus transmission.

Recent outbreaks have occurred in New Caledonia in 2011 (Dupont-Rouzeyrol et al., 2012), Papua New Guinea in 2012 (Horwood et al., 2013), Yap in 2013, Tonga in 2014, and French Polynesia in 2014. In December 2013, CHIKV was reported to cause autochthonous outbreaks for the first time in the Americas, Saint Martin Island, and the French West Indies (Leparc-Goffart et al., 2014). By March 2015, there are over 1,280,000 suspected cases, 26,000 confirmed cases, and 184 associated deaths as the disease spread to > 50 countries/territories in the Caribbean and the Americas, including the United States and Brazil (Pan American Health Organization 2015; Sam et al., 2015).

Indian Scenario

In India, the first CHIK outbreak occurred in 1963 in Kolkata (Shah et al., 1964), followed by epidemics in eastern coastal areas, namely Chennai, Pondicherry and Vellore in 1964, Visakhapatnam, Rajmundry and Kakinada in 1965 (Rao, 1966), Nagpur in 1965 (Rodrigues et al., 1972) and Barsi in 1973 (Padbidri & Gnaneswar,1979). In Chennai alone, nearly 400 000 cases were recorded in 1964. Chikungunya virus had almost disappeared from India after 1973 and since then no case was reported till the end of 2005. After a gap of 32 years, massive outbreaks of CHIK occurred during 2005–2006. Initially, two southern states (Andhra Pradesh and Karnataka) and one western state (Maharastra) were affected (Yergolkar et al., 2006). The outbreak was first investigated in February 2006 in Andhra Pradesh and then in March 2006 in Karnataka by health officials of the country who confirmed the occurrence of the chikungunya virus in the region. The number of suspected cases reported was up to a million. The outbreak has an attack rate of 4-45%. The outbreak continued with reports of a large number of cases from several other states including Rajasthan, Gujarat, Tamilnadu, Orrisa and Madhya Pradesh. A total of 129 districts in 8 states were affected by the virus (Cecilia, 2014). Genetic analysis revealed a novel ECSA genotype of CHIKV as the etiology of this unprecedented epidemic (Dash et al., 2007).

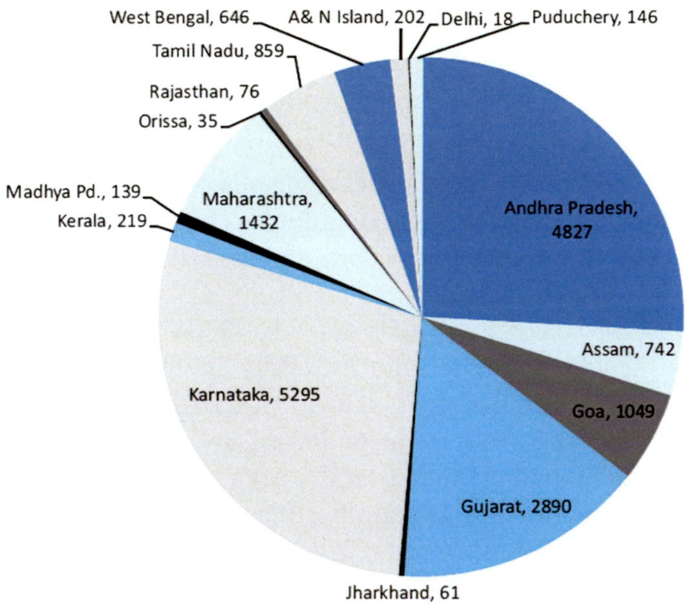

Figure 2.12: Distribution of chikungunya cases in Indian states in 2013 (based on NVBDCP data) http://nvbdcp.gov.in/chikun-status.html

Diagnosis

In humans, the Chikungunya fever (CHIKF) starts after 48 hours of the mosquito bite. A patient shows a high viremia load in their blood during 3-4 days of infection which declines during day 5-6 and disappears by day 7-8. Symptoms usually appear 4-7 days post-infection. Clinical manifestation of Chikungunya is very similar to those of Dengue fever hence the ability to distinguish CHIKV infection from dengue fever is a challenge in the areas where both the viruses simultaneously circulate (Carey, 1971). Virus isolation by culturing mosquito cells (C6/36), Vero cells or in mice (Couderc et al., 2008) is the most traditional and promising test for Chikungunya diagnosis. But the main disadvantages of this method are that it is time-consuming, requires handling of live viruses and shows high sensitivity only during the viremic phase. The Chikungunya confirmation can also be done by using gene amplification technologies viz; RT-PCR (Hasebe et al., 2002, Pfeffer et al., 2002; Pastorino et al., 2005; Edward et al., 2007; Joseph et al., 2008; Panning et al., 2009), Real-time RT-PCR (Carletti et al., 2007; Grivard et al., 2007; Laurent et al., 2007; Santhosh et al., 2007) and RT-LAMP (Parida et al., 2007). In these techniques, results could be available in 3-4 hours with the advantages of rapidity, lower contamination rate, higher sensitivity and higher specificity. But these techniques are very costly and requires sophisticated instrument and are hence unaffordable by most laboratories in resource-limited settings.

More frequently, serodiagnostic methods for the detection of immunoglobulin M (IgM) and immunoglobulin G (IgG) antibodies against CHIKV in acute and convalescent sera are used (Grivard et al., 2007). These include enzyme-linked immunosorbent assay (ELISA), indirect immunofluorescent method (Litzba et al., 2008), haemagglutination inhibition, or neutralization techniques. Thus in the majority of cases antibodies are being used for the diagnosis of CHIKV infection. The IgM antibody is detectable after a mean period of 3-4 days by ELISA and it persists for periods ranging from several weeks to 3 months. Instances of persistence of IgM antibodies 18 months after disease onset in about 40% of patients have also been described (Grivard et al., 2007; Borgherini et al., 2008).

The IgG antibodies can be detected in convalescent samples and persist for years. ELISA-based detection of CHIKV antigen has also been developed (Shukla et al., 2009; Kashyap et al., 2010; Kumar et al., 2012a; Khan et al., 2014). However, these assays are effective only for the early phase confirmation i.e. only 2-6 days after the onset of infection when the virus persists in the circulation. CHIKV IgM can be detected as early as 4 - 5 days after the onset of fever and persists for several months. So the detection of IgM antibodies against CHIKV would offer more window period for diagnosis of virus infection. In recent years, few commercial kits were launched in the market for the detection of Chikungunya virus but the sensitivity and specificity of these kits are poorly established and the possibility of false-positive results resulting from cross-reactivity with dengue virus or other arboviruses has to be considered (Rianthavorn et al., 2010; Blacksell et al., 2011).

The use of whole virus preparations as an antigen is associated with biohazards. CHIKV IgM ELISA based on the recombinant structural protein of virus expressed in baculovirus-infected insect cells has been reported (Cho et al., 2008 a; Cho et al., 2008 b). The early identification of patients at risk and treatment options for those with arthralgia are key areas for study. Although numerous methods for laboratory diagnosis have been developed in recent years, a significant unmet need is that of an affordable, simple, and reliable assay to be used in developing countries where CHIKV is mainly endemic (Sam et al., 2010).

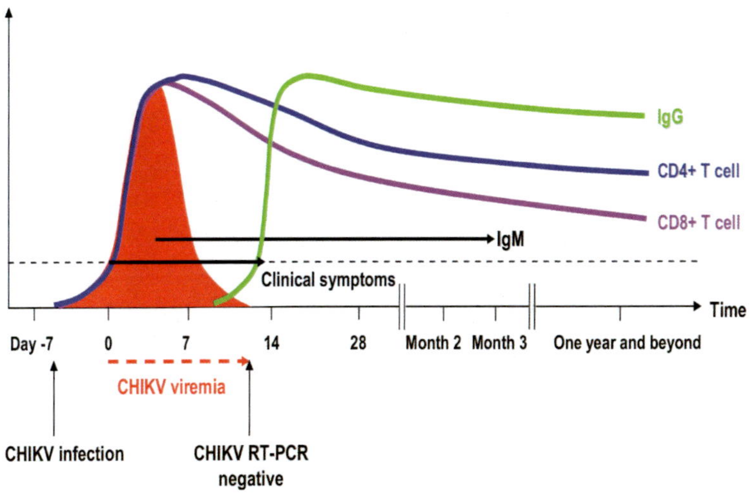

Figure 2.13: Schematic representation of immune response against CHIKV infection CHIKV viremia in blood lasts between 2 and 10 days (viral load in the red-filled area). Specific CD4þ (blue line) and CD8þ T cells (purple line) are expanded corresponding to CHIKV infection. Rapid virus elimination occurs before the expansion of neutralizing antibodies (IgG, green line), Clinical symptoms (fever) disappear when CHIKV viremia drops below the level of detection (Kam et al., 2009).

Clinical Manifestation and Symptoms

CHIKV initially replicates in the skin and disseminates to the liver and joints through the blood. Chikungunya virus infections in humans are associated with a range of clinical symptoms, such as high fever, headaches, rashes, myalgia, and arthralgia. The symptoms develop after an incubation period of 4-7 days. The disease is usually self-limiting and resolves in 1-2 weeks even without treatment. Rarely the symptoms may persist for a longer period and occasionally complications may develop. The occurrence of polyarthralgia along with myalgia is a typical feature of the illness. The joint pain is frightening in severity completely immobilizing many patients and can persist for several weeks or months. In 64% of patients, joint pain was reported even after 1 year of CHIKV post-infection. Female patients (100%) were significantly more likely to have persistent arthralgia than male patients (26.5%) (Chow et al., 2011; Win et al., 2010). The maculo popular and gingival hemorrhages are uncommon signs. Rashes occur mainly on trunks or extensor surfaces of the limbs and are itching in nature. Old age, prior joint pain, and underlying osteoarthritis co-morbidity were identified as risk factors for long-term rheumatic manifestations (Sam et al., 2015).

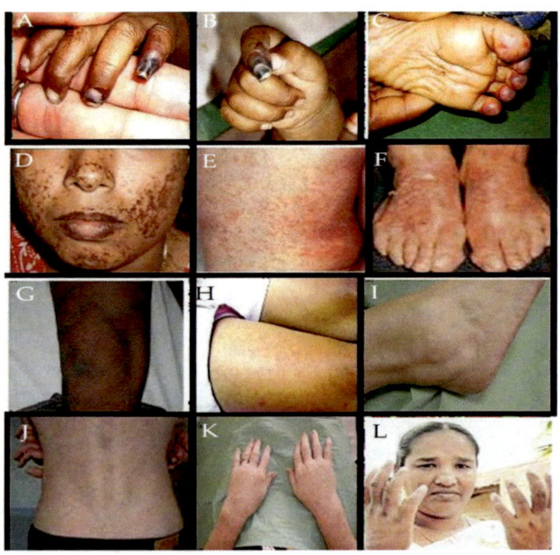

Figure 2.14: Symptoms associated with Chikungunya virus infection. Digital gangrene in an 8-month-old girl during week 3 of hospitalization. She was admitted to the hospital with fever, multiple seizures, and a widespread rash; chikungunya virus was detected in her plasma. A) Little finger of the left hand; B) index finger of the right hand; and C) 4 toes on the right foot. (Lewthwaite et al., 2009) Chikungunya-associated rheumatism second stage: (I) severe relapse

with polyarthritis and multiple tenosynovitis of wrists and fingers, (J) hypertrophic tenosynovitis at the ankle (Simon et al., 2008). (K) & (L) This rash appeared on the day of a febrile illness in a patient who presented with myalgia and arthralgia after visiting Mauritius (Photos by Richard Foster, South Africa).

Host Immune Response against Chikungunya Infection

Innate immune response

The potential of CHIKV to cause large epidemics and its expanding geographic range makes it necessary to understand the immune and pathogenic mechanisms active during the course of CHIKV infection in order to produce effective treatment and drugs. As soon as an infected mosquito bites the human the virus gets transmitted to the dermis of the skin and starts replicating at this site. Different cell types present in this site that actively plays role in innate immune response e.g. keratinocytes, macrophages, Langerhans cells and dendritic cells. The innate immune response gets activated as soon as any virus enters inside the cells. IFN system plays a major role in inhibiting virus spread at an early stage of infection (Schwartz and Albert, 2010).

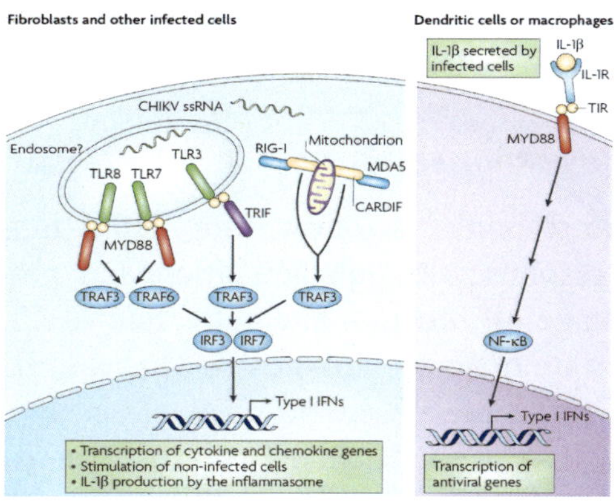

Figure 2.15: Innate immune control of chikungunya virus. (Schwartz and Albert, 2010).

Chikungunya virus (CHIKV) is a single-stranded RNA (ss RNA) virus and may generate double-stranded RNA intermediates during replication that have the potential to engage the pathogen recognition receptors Toll-like receptor 3 (TLR3), TLR7 and TLR8 and the retinoic acid-inducible gene I

(RIG-I)-like receptors (RLRs) melanoma differentiation-associated protein 5 (MDA5) and RIG-I. These receptors activate a signaling cascade that leads to the activation of type I interferons (IFNs) and the transcription of cytokines and chemokines. Recent evidence suggests that the production of type I IFNs by infected fibroblasts and other cell types is regulated by the adaptor protein CARDIF (CARD adaptor inducing IFNβ; also known as MAVS), which acts downstream of MDA5 and RIG-I. The inflammasome may also induce IL-1β production by infected cells. In a mouse model, protection was also partly dependent on the TLR adaptor myeloid differentiation primary response protein 88 (MYD88). This may suggest a role for TLRs, possibly on hematopoietic cells. In addition, MYD88 also acts as an adaptor for interleukin-1β receptor (IL-1R), which could be activated by the secretion of IL-1β from infected cells, thereby inducing type I IFN in non-infected cells. IRF, IFN regulatory factor; NF-κB, nuclear factor-κB; TIR, Toll/IL-1 receptor domain; TRAF, tumor necrosis factor receptor-associated factor; TRIF, TIR domain-containing adaptor protein inducing IFN-β. it is demonstrated that CHIKV infection in humans elicits strong innate immunity involving the production of numerous proinflammatory mediators. It has also been demonstrated that CHIKV antigens could be detected *in vivo* in the monocytes of acutely infected patients (Her et al., 2010). CHIKV interactions with monocytes, and with other blood leukocytes, induced a robust and rapid innate immune response with the production of specific chemokines and cytokines (Lum & Ng, 2015).

Adaptive immune response

The innate immune response is followed by activation of a more potent adaptive immune response through activation and proliferation of CD8 cells at an earlier stage of infection and activation of CD4 cells as well as production of proinflammatory cytokines IL-1RA and IL-2RA in the acute phase. The end of the acute phase is characterized by the production of IL-16, IL-17, IL-6, IL-8, CCL-5, MCP1, IP-10 by activated macrophages that are susceptible to CHIKV infection (Sourisseau et al., 2007). These chemokines help in the recruitment of monocytes, T cells and other effector molecules at the site of infection and help in the development of the antiviral defense. High plasma levels of type I IFNs, IL-4 and IL-7 cytokines that promote adaptive immunity suggest induction of a strong cellular immune response on infection with CHIKV (Gasque et al., 2015). The B cells promoting cytokines IL-4 and IL-10 upregulation at the first few days of onset of symptoms helps in the production of CHIKV-specific IgG. CD4+ T lymphocytes, which are also involved in the promotion of humoral responses, are strongly activated toward the end of the acute phase. IgG antibodies are detected in the first week after infection, indicating rapid seroconversion and high levels of antibody responses among CHIKV-infected individuals (Kam et al., 2012a; Gasque et al., 2015).

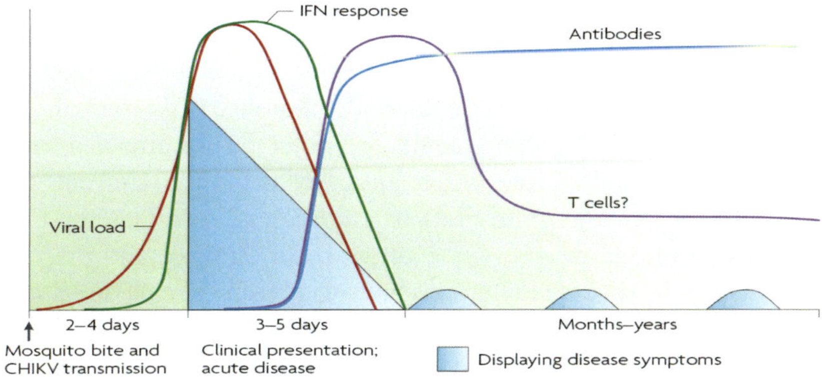

Figure 2.16: Chikungunya virus pathogenesis. Following transmission by mosquito bite, infected individuals experience an acute onset of disease 2–4 days after infection. Symptoms include high fever, rigors, headache and a petechial or maculopapular rash. In addition, most infected individuals complain of severe joint pain that is often incapacitating. Disease onset coincides with a rising viral titer, which triggers the activation of an innate immune response, the hallmark of which is the production of type I interferons (IFNs). Patients successfully clear the virus approximately 1 week after infection, and only at this time is their evidence of CHIKV-specific adaptive immunity (that is, T cell and antibody-mediated responses). Importantly, ~30% of individuals experience long-term sequellae that include arthralgia and, in some cases, arthritis. (Schwartz and Albert, 2010).

Control Measures

Due to the absence of a licensed vaccine, protection against mosquito bites and vector control are the main preventive measures. Breeding sites must be removed, destroyed, frequently emptied, and cleaned or treated with insecticides. Scale prevention campaigns using DDT have been effective against *A. aegypti* but not *A. albopictus*. Control of *A. aegypti* has rarely been achieved and never sustained (Reiter et al., 2006). Recent data show the different degrees of insecticide resistance in *A. albopictus* and *A. aegypti* (Cui et al., 2006). However, vector control is an endless, costly, and labor-intensive measure and is not always well accepted by local populations, whose cooperation is crucial.

CHIKV Vaccine Developments:

The spread of CHIKV could in theory be prevented by effective vector control. However, this has proven to be difficult (Weaver et al., 2012), which makes vaccination the most effective way of protecting humans and limiting further CHIKV transmission. CHIKV infection is believed to induce life-long immunity through a protective antibody response (Tiwari et al., 2009), indicating that naïve individuals could be protected for life if a safe and efficacious vaccine induces a similar antibody response. Currently, there are no specific treatments (antiviral) or commercial vaccines for CHIKV infections available. However, the emergence of CHIKV and the clinical manifestation of the disease in humans have triggered vaccine development. The first vaccine prototype was a formalin- inactivated virus, developed by the United States Army Medical Research Institute of Infectious Diseases (USAMRIID) (Harrison et al., 1971; Tiwari et al., 2009). Although efficacious, a major drawback is that production of the virus must take place in costly, biosafety level 3 facilities. As an alternative, live-attenuated virus vaccines have been developed (Levitt et al., 1986).

Live-attenuated virus vaccines have the advantage of inducing an efficient, balanced immune response, but have as a drawback the risk of reversion to virulence (Noad and Roy, 2003). The live-attenuated CHIKV vaccine (181/clone25) was tested in phase II clinical trials and elicited a protective immune response. However, 8% of tested volunteers developed transient arthralgia (Edelman et al., 2000). Although it is an effective vaccine candidate, the US Army has stopped further development of the attenuated vaccine strain (Weaver et al., 2012). Recent studies on the attenuated 181/clone25 CHIKV strain showed attenuation of the virus as a consequence of only two-point mutations, which were reversed in immunized mice. This clearly highlights the genetic instability of CHIKV attenuation (Gorchakov et al., 2012).

The prospect of live- (attenuated) alphavirus vaccine development remains questionable due to vaccine- induced clinical manifestations and the undeniable risk of transmission by mosquito vectors, but most critical is the possible reversion to virulence. In addition to the 181/clone25 vaccine, a broad range of vaccine strategies have been described (Table 2.1), including other live-attenuated virus vaccines (Levitt et al., 1986; Partidos et al., 2012;

Plante et al., 2011), chimeric virus vaccines (Wang et al., 2008), DNA vaccines (Muthumani et al., 2008; Mallilankaraman et al., 2011), adenoviral vectored vaccines (Wang et al., 2011), subunit protein vaccines (Kumar et al., 2012) and virus-like particles (VLP) formulations (Akahata et al., 2010). However, these vaccination strategies have their own specific complications in manufacturing, immunogenicity, safety, recombination and large-scale production (Edelman et al., 2000; Kutzler and Weiner, 2008). Recent studies have shown promising results in the development of a CHIKV VLP-based vaccine (Akahata et al., 2010).

The complete structural cassettes of different CHIKV strains were expressed via plasmid DNA transfection of 293T human kidney cells, there by producing CHIKV VLPs. Rhesus macaques were subsequently immunized with VLPs. The VLPs elicited a neutralizing antibody response against homologous and heterologous strains and protection against high-dose CHIKV challenge (Akahata et al., 2010). Regardless of the vaccine strategy, data obtained so far clearly showed that neutralizing antibodies play a major role in the protection against CHIKV infections (Weaver et al., 2012).

During natural infections, CHIKV induces high neutralizing antibody titers. The IgG antibodies are mainly directed against an N-terminal epitope on the exposed domain of E2 and to a lesser extent to E1, making them primary targets for subunit vaccine development (Vrati et al., 1988; Strauss & Strauss, 1991; Hunt et al., 2010; Kam et al., 2012b). The presence of the E2-directed IgG neutralizing antibodies correlates to long-term protection and viral clearance (Kam et al., 2012b; Kam et al., 2012c). To explore the potential of VLPs for the development of alphavirus in general, and CHIKV in particular, CHIKV-E1 and CHIKV-E2 were expressed as an individual subunits or expressed together with all CHIKV structural proteins as part of a VLP. This has been shown to be a safe and effective alternative to inactivated or attenuated live-virus formulations (Akahata et al., 2010; Kumar et al., 2012b) but is produced in a poorly scalable production system.

The production platform of choice should be safe to use, reach high production yields and be industrially scalable. The recombinant baculovirus-insect cell expression system serves as an elegant and safe production platform and has recently received wider attention for the large-scale production of VLP-based vaccine candidates against human viral disease (Vicente et al., 2011).

Table 2.1: Vaccine candidates against CHIKV infections (Ahola et al., 2015)

Strategy	Expression system	Antigen	Developmental stage
Inactivated virus	GMK-cells	Whole virus	Preclinical
Live-attenuated	GMK-cells	Whole virus	Terminated post clinical Phase II
DNA	pVax1 expression vector	C, E1, E2	Preclinical
Chimeric-vector	BHK-21-cells HEK-293-cells	C-E3-E2-6K-E1	Preclinical
IRES	Vero-cells	Whole virus	Preclinical
Subunit	Baculovirus	E1, E2	Preclinical
VLP subunit	293T-cells	C-E3-E2-6K-E1	Clinical Phase I
VLP subunit	Baculovirus	C-E3-E2-6K-E1	Preclinical

GMK-Green monkey kidney cells, BHK-Baby hamster kidney cells, HEK-Human embryonic kidney cells.

CHAPTER 3

DIFFERENT EXPRESSION SYSTEM TO GENERATE CHIKUNGUNYA VIRUS-LIKE PARTICLES

HETEROLOGOUS PLATFORM FOR RECOMBINANT PROTEIN PRODUCTION

Expression systems are normally referred to by the host that can express a desired foreign gene simultaneously with its own genes. Protein expression refers to the directed synthesis of large amounts of desired proteins. The heterologous production of proteins involves two major steps:

- Introduction of foreign DNA into the host cells. This step has three major considerations.
  - Identification and isolation of the DNA to be introduced
  - Identification of the vector and construction of recombinant vector
  - Identification of the suitable expression system to receive rDNA.
- Factors affecting the expression of foreign DNA for protein synthesis in the chosen expression system.

Prokaryotic and eukaryotic systems are the two general categories of expression systems. Prokaryotic systems are generally easier to handle and are satisfactory for most purposes. However, there are serious limitations in using prokaryotic cells for the production of eukaryotic proteins. For example, many of the eukaryotic proteins undergo a variety of post-translational modifications like proper folding, glycosylation, phosphorylation, formation of disulfide bridges, etc. There is no universal expression system for heterologous proteins. All expression systems have some advantages as well as some disadvantages that should be considered in selecting the right one. Choosing the best one requires evaluating the options from yield to glycosylation, to proper folding and to the economics of scale-up. Bacteria, yeast, mammalian and insect cells are generally used as expression hosts for the expression of recombinant viral proteins (Rai and Padh, 2001).

BACTERIAL EXPRESSION SYSTEM

E. coli is by far the most widely employed host. Its popularity is due to the vast body of knowledge about its genetics, physiology and complete genomic sequence which greatly facilitates gene cloning and cultivation (Shatzman and Rosenberg, 1987; Casadaban et al., 1983). High growth rates combined with the ability to express high levels of heterologous proteins make it an attractive host. *E. coli* can grow rapidly to high densities in simple and inexpensive media. Strains used for recombinant production have been genetically manipulated so that they are generally regarded as safe for large- scale fermentation. Purification has been greatly simplified by producing recombinant fusion proteins which can be affinity-purified (Maina et al., 1988). However, expression in bacteria does have some serious disadvantages. It poses significant problems in post- translational modifications of proteins. Common bacterial expression systems such as *E. coli* have no capacity to glycosylate proteins in either N- or O-linked conformation. The protein expressed in large amounts often precipitates into insoluble aggregates called inclusion bodies, from which it can only be recovered in an active form by solubilization in denaturing agents followed by careful renaturation (Marston et al., 1990). Lysis to recover the cytoplasmic proteins often results in the release of endotoxins, which must be removed from the final product. *E. coli* has toxic cell wall pyrogens and hence products need to be tested extensively before use (Makrides, 1996).

MAMMALIAN CELL EXPRESSION SYSTEM:

Ideally, proteins requiring mammalian post-translational modifications should be expressed in mammalian cells. If product authenticity is absolutely essential for clinical efficacy, then despite the many shortcomings, a mammalian host is the only choice, as it offers the greatest degree of product fidelity. It should, however, be noted that oligosaccharide processing is species- and cell type-dependent among mammalian cells. Differences in glycosylation patterns are reported in rodent cell lines and human tissues. Even the use of a human cell line is not perfect, since the transformation event required in most cases to produce a stable cell line may itself result in altered glycosylation profiles. Also, mammalian expression techniques are time-consuming and much more difficult to perform on a large scale. Complex nutrient requirements and low product concentrations have meant that the end product must bc highly value-added for this approach to be commercially viable (Kaufman et.al., 1990).

INSECT CELL EXPRESSION SYSTEM:

The baculoviruses have emerged as a popular system for over producing recombinant proteins in eukaryotic cells. Traditionally baculovirus expression systems are based on an *in vivo* low-frequency recombination event between a shuttle vector carrying the gene of interest and the circular *Autographa californica* nuclear polyhedrosis virus (AcNPV) double-stranded DNA viral genome. Several factors have contributed to their popularity. The baculovirus expression system is a potent eukaryotic expression that can be utilized to express a variety of recombinant proteins at levels as high as 500 mg per liter (O'Reilly et al., 1992). Being eukaryotes, they use many of the protein modifications, processing, and transport systems present in higher eukaryotic cells (O'Reilly et al., 1992). Insect cells possess similar post-translational modification as mammalian cells. These post-translational modifications include phosphorylation, glycosylation, myristolation and palmitolation. They use a helper-independent virus that can be propagated to high titers in insect cells adapted for growth in suspension cultures, making it possible to obtain large amounts of recombinant proteins with relative ease. Expressed proteins are usually expressed in the proper cellular compartment, i.e. membrane proteins are usually localized to the membrane, nuclear proteins to the nucleus, and secreted proteins secreted into the medium. The majority of the over produced proteins remain soluble, correctly folded and biologically active in insect cells. Since the genome of AcNPV is large (130 kb) and thus can accommodate large fragments of foreign DNA.

Baculoviruses are non-infectious to vertebrates and their promoters have been shown to be inactive in mammalian cells, which gives them a possible advantage over other systems when expressing oncogenes or potentially toxic proteins. Also, the process development time is short. Expression using baculoviral vectors also has some limitations. Since baculoviruses infect invertebrates, it is possible that the processing of proteins produced by vertebrates is different and this seems to be the case for some post-translational modifications, e.g. internal proteolytic cleavages at arginine- or lysine-rich sequences are highly inefficient. The glycosylation capability is generally limited to producing only high mannose type and not processed to complex type oligosaccharides containing fructose, galactose and sialic acid. Also, the insect cell expression system is a slow-growing system, growing on complex media which raises its economic cost (Rueda et al., 2000).

YEAST EXPRESSION SYSTEM

Yeast is the favored alternative host for the expression of foreign proteins for research, industrial or medicinal use (Hitzeman et. al., 1981). As a food organism, it is highly acceptable for the production of pharmaceutical proteins. In contrast, *E. coli* has toxic cell wall pyrogens and mammalian cells may contain oncogenic or viral DNA. Compared to mammalian cells, yeast can be grown relatively rapidly (doubling time 90 min) on simple media and to high cell density and its genetics is more advanced than any other eukaryote so that it can be manipulated readily. Added advantages are the availability of complete genomic sequence, the nuclear stable high copy plasmids and the ability to secrete the target protein (Hitzeman et al., 1990). These lower eukaryotic systems are able to glycosylate the target proteins, but it has been shown that both N- and O-linked oligosaccharide structures are, however, significantly different from their mammalian counterparts (Kornfeld et al, 1985; Kukuruzinska et al., 1987). Hypermannosylation (addition of a large number of mannose residues to the core oligosaccharide) is a common feature in yeast, hindering proper folding and therefore the activity of the protein. At the moment yeast provides a good compromise between bacteria on one side and mammalian cell lines on the other.

Table-3.1: Comparison of expression system (Lundstrom et al., 2006; Byrne, 2015)

Desired characteristics	**Expression system**			
	Bacteria	**Yeast**	**Insect cell**	**Mammalian cell**
Cell growth	Rapid	Rapid	Slow	Slow
Complexity of growth Medium	Minimum	Minimum	Complex	Complex
Cost of growth Medium	Low	Low	High	High
Expression level	High	Low to High	Low to High	Low to moderate
Extracellular Expression	Secretion to periplasm	Secretion to medium	Secretion to medium	Secretion to medium
Post transitional Modifications				
Protein folding	Refolding usually required	Refolding may be required	Proper folding	Proper folding
N-linked Glycosylation	None	High mannose	Simple, no sialic acid	Complex
O- linked Glycosylation	No	Yes	Yes	Yes
Phosphorylation	No	Yes	Yes	Yes
Acetylation	No	Yes	Yes	Yes
Acylation	No	Yes	Yes	Yes
γ – Carboxylation	No	No	No	Yes

PICHIA PASTORIS EXPRESSION SYSTEM FOR THE BULK PRODUCTION OF VACCINES

Features of Pichia Pastoris

The production of recombinant proteins is intimately related to the cellular machinery of the producer microorganism. For the last two decades, *E. coli* has been the "factory" of choice for the expression of many heterologous proteins. However, *E. coli* is a prokaryote and lacks intracellular organelles needed for post-translational modifications. Therefore, researchers have recently inclined to eukaryotic yeast *Pichia pastoris* (Cregg et al., 2000). *Pichia pastoris* is a highly successful system for the production of a wide variety of recombinant proteins. It is a single-celled microorganism that is easy to manipulate and culture as *E.coli*.

Pichia pastoris (*P. pastoris*) is a methylotrophic yeast, capable of metabolizing methanol as a sole carbon source. That has emerged as a viable recombinant protein production system for the biotechnology and pharmaceutical industries. It can use a strong methanol inducible promoter of alcohol oxidase 1 (AOX1) for protein expression. It is capable of producing high levels of therapeutic recombinant proteins up to the order of grams per liter. However, recombinant protein expression levels in *P. pastoris* are highly protein specific. High-level production may be obtained for one type of protein, but a very low level is obtained for another type of protein. The range has been observed to be as wide as from 20 mg/L to 14.8 g/L (Romanos et al., 1992).

The AOX Promoter

An essential element required for any expression system is a strong promoter to drive the expression of a foreign gene. In *Pichia pastoris* it is the AOX promoter that encodes for the alcohol oxidase (AOX) enzyme. AOX is an oligomeric octamer flavoprotein. Its every subunit contains one noncovalently bound FAD (flavin adenine di-nucleotide). Alcohol oxidase has a poor affinity for oxygen so the methylotrophic yeast has to synthesize this enzyme in large amounts for the oxidation of alcohols. The AOX is not specific to methanol and can oxidize other primary alcohols. However, as the number of carbon in the alcohol increases, the activity of the enzyme decreases. There are two genes in *Picia pastoris* that code for alcohol oxidase, AOX1 and AOX2 but the AOX1 gene is responsible for the majority alcohol oxidase activity in the cell. The expression of the AOX gene is tightly regulated; it is strongly repressed by many alternate carbon sources such as glucose and glycerol and is induced by carbon starvation and high methanol levels. The presence of methanol is essential to induce high levels of transcription (Cregg et al., 2000). In methanol-grown shake flask cultures, it has been seen that the level of AOX1 is typically 5 % of total soluble protein but can be more than 30% in a fed-batch fermentor culture. The expression of the AOX gene is controlled at the level of transcription (Cregg et al., 1987). In methanol growing cells, AOX1 mRNA can comprise up to approximately 5 % of the total polyA-RNA pool where as cells grown on other carbon sources have an undetectable amount of AOX1 mRNA (Cregg et al., 1993).

Table 3.2: Advantages and disadvantages of using AOX1 promoter (Cregg et al., 1993; Cereghino et al., 2000)

Advantages	Disadvantages
Transcription of the foreign protein is tightly regulated and controlled by repression/derepression mechanism.	Monitoring methanol during a process is often difficult, due to the unreliability of on-line probes and the complications of measuring off-line.
High levels of foreign proteins can be expressed, even if they are toxic to the cell.	Methanol is a fire hazard; therefore, storing the large quantities required for these processes is undesirable.
The repression of transcription by the initial carbon source ensures that good cell growth is obtained before the gene product is overexpressed.	Methanol is mainly derived from petrochemical sources, which may be unsuitable for use in the production of certain food products and additives.
Induction of transcription is easily achieved by the addition of methanol.	Two carbon sources are required, with a switching over from one to the other at a precise time point.

Methanol Metabolism in *Pichia*

Methylotrophic yeasts have four genera, *Candida, Hansenula, Tourulopsis and Pichia*. The methanol metabolizing pathway in all methylotrophic yeast appears to be the same. The first step in methanol metabolism is the oxidation of methanol to formaldehyde by the enzyme alcohol oxidase (AOX). In this process, hydrogen peroxide is generated, which is toxic to cells. Since this process takes place within a specialized organelle, called peroxisome, which converted H_2O_2 to H_2O and O_2 by peroxisome catalase enzyme. The presence of hydrogen peroxide producing oxidases and catalase is a characteristic feature of peroxisomes in all eukaryotes and has the advantage that the enzymes that produce and decompose hydrogen peroxide are closely associated, preventing diffusion of this hazardous compound into the cytoplasm (Werten et al., 1999).

The conversion of methanol to formaldehyde by alcohol oxidase is the rate-limiting step in utilizing methanol and is regulated by increasing the amount of the AOX enzyme in the cell. The formaldehyde is then further oxidized either through a cytosolic dissimilatory pathway, which yields energy or an assimilatory pathway for the generation of biomass. In the dissimilatory pathway, a portion of the formaldehyde generated by AOX leaves the peroxisome and is further oxidized to formate and carbon dioxide by two cytoplasmic dehydrogenases (FLD and FMDH), reactions that are a source of energy for cells growing on methanol. In the assimilatory pathway, the remaining formaldehyde is assimilated to form cellular constituents by a cyclic pathway that starts with the condensation of formaldehyde with xylulose 5-monophosphate, a reaction catalyzed by a third peroxisomal enzyme dihydroxyacetone synthase (DHAS). The products of this reaction, glyceraldehyde 3-phosphate and dihydroxyacetone, leave the peroxisome and enter a cytoplasmic pathway that regenerates xylulose 5-monophosphate and, for every three cycles, one net molecule of glyceraldehyde 3- phosphate is generated (Cereghino & Cregg, 2000).

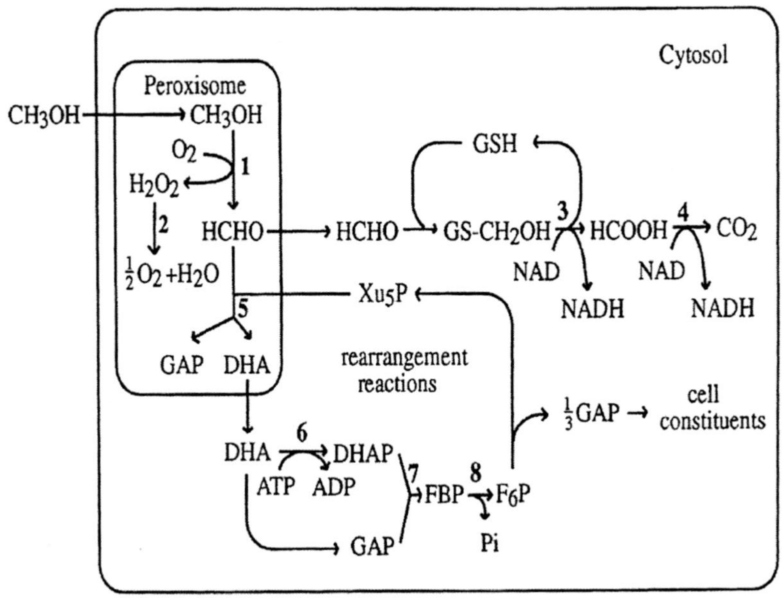

Figure 3.1: The methanol pathway in *P. pastoris*.1, Alcohol oxidase; 2, catalase; 3, formaldehyde dehydrogenase; 4, formate dehydrogenase, 5, dihydroxyacetone synthase; 6, dihydroxyacetone kinase; 7, fructose 1,6-biphosphate aldolase; 8, fructose 1,6- bisphosphatase (Cereghino & Cregg, 2000).

Expression Vectors of *Pichia Pastoris*

Plasmid vectors designed for heterologous protein expression in *P. pastoris* have several common features. The foreign gene expression cassette is one of those and is composed of DNA sequences containing the *P. pastoris* *AOX1* promoter, followed by one or more unique restriction sites for insertion of the foreign gene, followed by the transcriptional termination sequence from the *P. pastoris AOX1* gene that directs efficient 3' processing and polyadenylation of the mRNAs. Some vectors also contain *AOX1* 3' flanking sequences that are derived from a region of the *P. pastoris* genome that lies immediately 3' of the *AOX1* gene and can be used to direct fragments containing a foreign gene expression cassette to integration at the *AOX1* locus by gene replacement (or gene insertion 3' to *AOX1* gene). Additional features that are present in certain *P. pastoris* expression vectors serve as tools for specialized functions. For the secretion of foreign proteins, vectors have been constructed that contain a DNA sequence immediately following the *AOX1* promoter that encodes a secretion signal.

The most frequently used of these is the *S. cerevisiae* α factor pre pro signal sequence. However, vectors containing the signal sequence derived from the *P. pastoris* acid phosphatase gene (*PHO1*) are also available. Vectors with dominant drug resistance markers that allow for enrichment of strains that receive multiple copies of foreign gene expression cassettes during transformations have been developed. One set of vectors (pPIC3K and pPIC9K) contains the bacterial kanamycin-resistance gene and confers resistance to high levels of G418 upon strains that contain multiple copies of these vectors. Another set of vectors, the pPICZ series, contains the *Sh ble* gene from *Streptoalloteichus hindustanus*. This gene is small (375 bp) and confers resistance to the drug Zeocin in *E. coli*, yeasts (including *P. pastoris*) and other eukaryotes. Because the *Sh ble* gene serves as the selectable marker for both *E. coli* and *P. pastoris*, the ZeoR vectors are much smaller (~3 kb) and easier to manipulate than other *P. pastoris* expression vectors. These vectors also contain a multiple cloning site (MCS) with several unique restriction sites for the convenience of foreign gene insertion and sequences encoding the His6 and *myc* epitopes so that foreign proteins can be easily epitope-tagged at their carboxyl termini, if desired. Another feature present on certain vectors (e.g., pAO815 and the pPICZ vector series) is designed to facilitate the construction of expression vectors with multiple expression cassette copies. Multiple copies of an expression cassette are introduced in these vectors by inserting an expression cassette bounded by a *Bam*HI and a *Bgl*II site into the *Bam*HI site of a vector already containing a single expression cassette copy. The resulting *Bam*HI/*Bgl*II junction between the two cassettes can no longer be cleaved by either enzyme allowing for the insertion of another *Bam*HI-*Bgl*II-bounded cassette into the same vector to generate a vector with three cassette copies. The process of addition is repeated until six to eight copies of a cassette are present in a single final vector, which is then transformed into the

P. pastoris host strain. Finally, vectors containing a constitutive *P. pastoris* promoter derived from the *P. pastoris* glyceraldehyde-3-phosphate dehydrogenase gene (*GAP*) have recently become available. The *GAP* promoter is a convenient alternative to the *AOX1* promoter for the expression of genes whose products are not toxic to *P. pastoris*. In addition, its use does not involve the use of methanol, which may be problematic in some instances (Cregg et al., 2000; Romans, 1995)

Advantages of *Pichia Pastoris* as an Expression Host

As an outstanding host for the production of recombinant proteins, it offers many other advantages. Since the proteins produced in *P. pastoris* are typically folded correctly, the fermentation of genetically engineered *P. pastoris* provides an excellent alternative to *E. coli* expression systems (Jahic et al., 2003). *Pichia pastoris* has a prolific growth rate and can be grown to very high cell densities (Jahic et al., 2003). However, in a batch mode, the growth of the cells is limited by the nutrients present in the medium at the time of inoculation. A fed-batch system enables to control the addition of just enough methanol for protein synthesis while preventing excess methanol addition which can cause toxicity (Romanos, 1995).

Pichia pastoris has emerged as an ideal organism to express viral antigens because yeast glycosylates proteins more similar to mammals than bacteria. Compared with insect or mammalian cells, the expression of recombinant proteins in yeast could present a viable alternative in terms of large-scale vaccine production and a short time-line suitable for rapid response in an influenza pandemic. Multiple copy integration of recombinant genes in *Pichia* has been demonstrated to increase the expression of the desired protein in many cases (Cregg et al., 1993; Scorer et al., 1994). More recently, *P. pastoris* has been used to express therapeutic proteins that have entered clinical trials (Gerngross 2004; Byrne, 2015).

Further development in the field of therapeutic glycoprotein production with *P. pastoris* strains is expected due to recent advances in genetic engineering of human glycosylation pathways into yeasts (Choi et al., 2003; Bobrowicz et al., 2004). With the ability to replicate certain human glycosylation patterns, yeast-based expression platforms offer an attractive alternative to current mammalian or insect cell culture processes due to a variety of additional advantages *viz* cheaper operating costs, simple chemically defined media and no viral contamination.

Disadvantages of *Pichia Pastoris*

Foreign proteins secreted from *P. pastoris* receive much more carbohydrates and appear by SDS-PAGE and western blotting to be hyperglycosylated. Interestingly, *P. pastoris* does not appear to be capable of adding α1,3-terminal mannose to oligosaccharides. This contrasts with *S. cerevisiae* oligosaccharides where α1,3-linked terminal mannose is common. N-linked high mannose oligosaccharides added to proteins by *Pichia pastoris* represent a significant problem in the use of foreign secreted proteins by the pharmaceutical industry. They can be exceedingly antigenic when introduced intravenously into mammals and are rapidly cleared from the blood by the liver (Cregg et al., 2000).

Different Foreign Proteins Produced in *Pichia Pastoris*

The *Pichia* expression system has been widely used to produce a variety of different heterologous proteins. Since 2002 there has been a great increase in foreign protein production in *Pichia*. Cell growth is particularly important for secreted protein production in bioreactors since the concentration of the product in the extracellular medium is roughly proportional to the concentration of cells in the culture in many instances. The yields of proteins expressed intracellularly in bioreactors are also high, due to the efficiency of the *AOX1* promoter (Cereghino & Cregg, 2000). Production of large amounts of heterologous proteins in shake-flask culture is difficult, due to the limitations of volume, oxygen transfer, substrate addition and an inability to monitor these factors efficiently. Methods of monitoring methanol in shake flasks are available, such as organic solvent vapor detectors (Guarna et al., 1997), and the oxygen transfer of these systems can be increased by the use of baffles (Villatte et al., 2001). On-line measurement of oxygen and carbon dioxide transfer rates in shake flasks has also been demonstrated using a respiration activity monitoring system (RAMOS) (Silberbach et al., 2003). However, the use of bioreactors is preferable, since all of these parameters can be monitored and controlled simultaneously, allowing more efficient production of the desired heterologous protein (Macauley-Patrick et al., 2005).

Table 3.3: Production of different viral proteins in *P. pastoris* (Cregg et al., 2000; Byrne, 2015)

Protein	**Comments: mode, amount, signal sequence**
Hepatitis B virus surface antigen	I, 400 mg l^{-1}
Human immunodeficiency virus type 1 (HIV-1)envelope glycoprotein, gp120 (ENV)	S, 20 mg l^{-1}, α-MF
Hepatitis B virus surface antigen-HIV gp41 epitope chimera	I
Bovine herpes virus-1 glycoprotein D	S, 20 mg l^{-1}, α-MF
Dengue virus type 1 structural gene recombinant E protein	S, PHO1, prM virus signal sequence
Hepatitis E virus ORF3	I
Polyomavirus large T antigen	I, 0.5 mg l^{-1}
Reovirus lambda 1 core protein	I, 0.8 mg l^{-1}
Vaccinia virus complement control protein	S, 3 mg l^{-1}, α-MF
Reovirus sigma 1 protein	I
A/VICTORIA/3/75 in£uenza virus neuraminidase head domain	S, 3 mg ml^{-1}, α-MF
Human papillomavirus type 16 and 18 capsid protein (L1)	I
Reticuloendotheliosis virus gp90 protein	S, 100 mg l^{-1}
H1N1 haemagglutinin protein	S, 430 mg l^{-1}, α-MF
Avian influenza A (H5N1) virus haemagglutinin protein	I
Equine Infectious Anemia Virus (EIAV) Antigen	S, 230μg ml^{-1}

I = intracellular (with subcellular location), S=secreted, Signal sequences: α-MF (S. cerevisiae α-mating factor); PHO1 (*P. pastoris* acid phosphatase)

CHAPTER 4

METHODS TO DEVELOP CHIK-VLPS

INTRODUCTION

VIRUSES

Chikungunya virus (ECSA E1: A226 V isolate, DRDE07 GenBank accession number EU372006) isolated from an infected patient during the 2007 outbreak in Kerala, India [East-Central-South- African (ECSA) genotype] and maintained in the Division of Virology, Defence research and development establishment (DRDE), Gwalior was used as the reference standard in the assay systems. This virus was used at passage level 10 in Vero cells in the present study. Some of the representative members of the Flavivirus group *viz*.; the four dengue virus serotypes (DEN-1, Hawaii; DEN-2, ThNH7/93; DEN-3, PhMH-J1-97; DEN-4, SLMC 318), Japanese Encephalitis virus (JEV) JaOArS982 strain and Yellow fever virus, were used in the present study for checking the cross-reactivity. All the live virus experiments were performed at the BSL-3 facility, DRDE, Gwalior.

Bacterial Strains and Vectors

Escherichia coli (DH5-α) procured from Invitrogen, USA, was initially used for transforming the chimeric recombinant construct. The yeast transfer vector pPIC9K and pTZ57 vector (Invitrogen, USA) were used for the initial cloning of the CHIKV polyprotein gene

Yeast Strain

The *Pichia pastoris* yeast strain GS115 obtained from Molecular Virology laboratory, Indian Veterinary Research Institute, Bangalore was used in the present study.

Media, Chemicals, and Solutions

All the chemicals were purchased from Sigma (USA) and Himedia (India). Viral RNA mini kit, QIAquick Gel Extraction Kit was from Qiagen (Hilden, Germany). RT- PCR kit, Antibody isotyping kit, kanamycin, Fluorescein isothiocyanate (FITC)- conjugated anti-mouse goat antibodies and all secondary antibody–enzyme conjugates (anti-mouse, anti-rabbit, anti-human horseradish peroxidase) were from Sigma (USA). Restriction enzymes, T4 DNA Ligase, 1000 bp and 100 bp DNA ladders, Protein molecular weight markers, 6X loading dye for agarose gel electrophoresis were from MBI Fermentas (Hanover, MD, USA). BD OptEIA Cytokine profiling Kit was procured from BD Biosciences, USA. ABI PRISM Big Dye® terminator v3.1cycle sequencing ready reaction kit (Applied Biosystems, USA). The composition of buffers and reagents used in the present study is given in the appendix.

Glasswares and Plastic Wares

Glasswares were purchased from Borosil (India) and Schott-Duran (Germany). Plasticwares were procured from Greiner Bio-One (Austria), Tarsons products Pvt. Ltd. (India), Axygen (USA) and Nunc International Corporation, Denmark.

ANIMALS AND ETHICS STATEMENT

Four weeks old Balb/c mice, 4 days old neonatal Balb/c mice and 6–8 weeks old rabbit (New Zealand white strain) were used in the study. All the animals were obtained from the Animal facility, DRDE, Gwalior. The animal studies experiments had approval from the Institutional Animal Ethics Committee (IAEC) approved by Defence Research Development & Establishment (DRDE), India vide registration number 37/1999/CPCSEA (Committee for the purpose of control and supervision on experiments on animals), Ministry of Social Justice, Government of India and adopted by the Institutional Biosafety Committee (IBSC). Animals were maintained in accordance with the recommendations of the committee for the purpose of control and supervision of experiments on animals, Govt. of India. The food and water were provided *ad libitum* and the principles of good laboratory animal care were followed all through the experimental process. The animal studies were conducted in a biosafety level-3 containment facility, following the standard operating procedures for the facility. After experiments were performed, all animals were euthanized by anesthesia with CO2 and collected whole blood from the heart.

Clinical Samples

A panel of 100 serum samples including 40 Chikungunya suspected clinical samples, 20 Dengue and 20 JE infected patent sera samples and 20 healthy persons sera samples was included in this study. 40 CHIKV suspected clinical samples were collected from Byramjee Jeejeebhoy Government Medical College, Pune, India, from September 2014 to November 2014 and stored at −80°C until they were used. The cross-reactivity study was also attempted with a panel of serum samples obtained from healthy persons in addition to the samples from dengue and Japanese encephalitis (Dash et al., 2006; Dash et al. 2007).

Cell Culture

Vero cells (African green monkey kidney cells) were used for virus maintenance, propagation and titration. This cell line was obtained from National Centre for Cell Science (NCCS) in Pune, India. Vero cells were maintained in Eagles Minimum essential medium (EMEM), supplemented with 10% (v/v) fetal bovine serum (FBS), in a 5% CO_2 humidified incubator, at 37°C.

Virus Propagation

Chikungunya virus (CHIKV) was maintained in Vero cell lines. CHIKV was repeatedly passaged on the Vero cell line to increase the viral titer. The viral titer was determined by plaque assay. Thus produced high titered virus was raised in bulk volume in Vero cells. Briefly, African green monkey kidney (V*ero*) cells were cultured in four T- 175 cm^2 cell culture flasks (Greiner, USA) at 37°C, 5% CO2 in Dulbecco's modified Eagle's medium (Sigma, USA) supplemented with 10% heat-inactivated fetal bovine serum (FBS) (Sigma, USA) and 100 units of penicillin and 100 µg/ml streptomycin. Cells were grown to 90% confluency and were infected with CHIKV at a multiplicity of infection (m.o.i.) of 1. CHIKV was then allowed to adsorb on the surface of cells for 90 minutes at 37°C. After incubation, the unabsorbed virus was removed by washing with PBS and cells were further incubated with fresh DMEM with 2% FBS. After infection, fresh medium containing 2% of FBS was added to the cells and the cells were incubated at 37°C, 5% CO_2 until cytopathic changes were observed. The virus was harvested after observing cytopathic changes in the cell monolayer and stored at -80°C. On thawing, the infected cell suspensions were clarified by centrifugation at 3000 x g for 20 min at 4°C using a centrifuge (Sigma, USA).

Plaque Assay

The plaque assay was performed in Vero cells using a modified protocol from Roehrig et al., 2008. Briefly, the cells were seeded in a 24-well plate to almost 90% confluency and a density of 4 $x10^5$ cells /well and incubated overnight at 37^{0}C in 5% CO_2. The medium was removed from cells and replaced with 200ml of medium containing 10-fold serially diluted CHIKV. Virus adsorption was allowed to proceed for 90 min at 37°C with rocking of the plate every 15 min. Then the cells were washed with PBS and overlaid with 1ml/well of MEM containing 2% FBS and 1.25% methyl cellulose (Sigma, USA). Plates were incubated at 37°C in 5% CO_2 for 3 days and the overlay media was removed after 3 days and cells were fixed with chilled methanol for 1 hr. The fixed cell monolayers were stained with 0.8% crystal violet. Subsequently, plates were rinsed and dried at room temperature, and plaques were counted immediately. Every time the assay was carried out in duplicate and the plaque counts were averaged. The viral titers were expressed as plaque-forming units (PFU)/ml, calculated as PFU/ml: [(number of plaques per well) x (dilution)]/(inoculum volume).

Virus Concentration

The clarified viral supernatant was subsequently concentrated by adding 50% (w/v) PEG 6000 in NT buffer (100 mM NaCl, 50 mM Tris-HCl, pH 7.2) to a final concentration of 20% (v/v). The virus particles were then precipitated for 3 hrs. at 4°C with moderate stirring on a magnetic stirrer, followed by centrifugation at 8000 × g for 30 min at 4°C in a Sorvall centrifuge. The supernatant was removed and the pellet was then re-suspended in 2ml of ice-cold NT buffer.

Chikungunya Virus Purification by Ultracentrifugation

Discontinuous sucrose gradients were prepared by sequentially layering 60 and 20% sucrose solution (w/v in TNE buffer) into 13 ml centrifuge tubes (Thermo scientific, USA), and the gradients were used immediately. PEG-6000 concentrated virus samples were layered over a discontinuous sucrose gradient and centrifuged in a TH-641 swinging bucket rotor (Thermo Scientific, USA) for 16 hrs at 35,000 rpm at 4°C. The gradient fractions along with the opaque band at 20-60% interface were harvested separately. The presence of Chikungunya virus in fraction samples was determined by SDS-PAGE, western blotting, reverse transcription polymerase chain reaction and finally by TEM as described below.

SDS-PAGE Analysis of Purified CHIKV

The fractions collected after ultra centrifugation were analyzed by 10% sodium dodecyl sulfate polyacrylamide gel electrophoresis (SDS-PAGE) and visualized by Coomassie staining (Laemmli, 1970). The procedure followed is as described below; SDS-PAGE was carried out with a discontinuous buffer system with a 10% separating gel (pH 8.8) and 5% resolving gel (pH 6.8) of 1mm thickness. The plates were fixed using clips at the sides and agar at the bottom. The resolving gel (10%) was prepared by mixing water, 30% Acrylamide, 1.5M Tris pH 8.8, 10% SDS, 10% APS and TEMED. Water saturated Methanol was added over the gel. The resolving gel was allowed to polymerize after which the methanol was poured off and the gel was rinsed with distilled water and dried with filter paper. The stacking gel (5%) was prepared by mixing water, 30% Acrylamide, 1M Tris pH 6.8, 10% SDS, 10% APS and TEMED and was poured above the resolving gel. The comb was placed and allowed the gel to get polymerize. The gel after polymerizing was transferred into an electrophoretic apparatus (Bio-Rad, USA) and the buffer chambers were filled with running buffer (Appendix). The protein samples were mixed with sample buffer/loading buffer (Appendix) and were loaded into the wells of the gel along with a standard protein molecular weight marker. The gel was subjected to electrophoresis at 70V till the tracking dye reached the separating gel. The voltage was increased to 100V and continued till the dye front reached the bottom of the separating gel. After completion of electrophoresis, the gel was stained with 0.25% (w/v) coomassie Brilliant Blue (CBB-R 250) in 45:10:45:methanol/Acetic acid/water for 10 hours and destained with regular changing of the destaining solution (10% v/v acetic acid and 40% methanol solution in water for 5-6 hours). The gel was visualized on a white illuminator. The gel was stored in 5% acetic acid containing a few drops of glycerol. Molecular weights of the proteins were determined based on relative mobilities (Sharpio et al., 1967).

Western Blot Analysis of Purified CHIKV

The same fractions were also subjected to western blotting using in-house mouse polyclonal antibodies raised against recombinant Chikungunya E2 protein. In brief, after SDS-PAGE the gel was equilibrated for 5 minutes in transfer buffer (48 mM Tris base, 39 M glycine, 20% methanol, pH 9.2). For western blot, the gel having the purified fractions along with molecular weight marker was then placed over an activated Poly vinyl difluoride (PVDF) membrane assembled on Trans-blot semidry transfer cell unit (Bio-Rad, USA) and 50mA current was applied for 1 hour. The membrane was blocked overnight at 4^0C in 10 ml blocking buffer. The blot was washed with 0.05% PBST thrice for 5 min and incubated with mouse polyclonal antibodies raised against recombinant Chikungunya E2 protein for 1 h at 37^0C. The blots were then thoroughly washed thrice with PBST for 5 min each followed by incubation with 10 ml of 1:3000 anti-mouse horse raddish peroxidase conjugated IgG (Sigma, USA) as secondary antibodies for 60 min. The blot was washed 5 times for 2 min each in PBST. The color development was done using H_2O_2/DAB substrate/chromogen (Sigma, USA) for 5 min and the blot was washed with an excess of distilled water to stop the reaction. The results obtained were documented.

Viral RNA Extraction

The viral RNA was extracted from CHIKV infected culture supernatant using the QIAamp viral RNA mini kit (Qiagen, Germany), according to the manufacturer's protocol, as described. 140 μl of infected culture supernatant was added to 560 μl of buffer AVL and the mixture was incubated at room temperature for 10 min. 560 μl of ethanol was added to the mixture and vortexed for 5 sec. 630 μl of this mixture was then carefully applied to the QIAamp spin column (placed inside a 2 ml collection tube) and centrifuged at 8000 rpm for 1 min. The filtrate was discarded. The remaining 630 μl of this mixture was applied to the above column and the column was again centrifuged at 8000 rpm for 1 min. The spin column was placed on a new collection tube and washed with 500 μl of buffer AW1 and 500 μl of buffer AW2 respectively. The spin column was again placed in a fresh 2ml collection tube and centrifuged at 13000 rpm for 2 min. to remove any residual wash buffer. The column was then placed in a new DEPC treated 1.5 ml Eppendorf tube. 30 µl of AVE elution buffer was applied to the center of the column and centrifuged at 8000 rpm for 1 min. This step was repeated and finally, the eluted RNA (around 60 µl) was stored at –70^{0}C.

CONFIRMATION OF PURIFIED CHIKUNGUNYA VIRUS THROUGH REVERSE TRANSCRIPTION POLYMERASE CHAIN REACTION (RT-PCR)

The genetic identity of the Chikungunya virus after purification was confirmed by reverse transcription polymerase chain reaction (RT-PCR). Genomic RNA was extracted from the purified virus after ultracentrifugation. The region encoding the partial CHIKV polyprotein was further amplified by RT-PCR using specific primers to confirm the genetic identity of the purified virus.

Table 4.1: Primer sequences and the characteristics of CHIKV structural polyprotein specific amplicon

S.No.	Primer Code	Primer sequence (restriction site underlined)	Product size (Kb)
1.	**CHIKYVLP MFWD (*Xho* I)**	5'- TGA AGG GCT CGA GGT CAC GTG - 3' (Base pair + 9520 to + 9533 Gene bank: EU372006.1)	1.795 Kbp
2.	**CHIKYVLP REV (*Avr* II)**	5'-TA CCTAGGTTA TTA TTC TTA GTG CCT GCT G -3' (Base pair + 11313 to + 11301 Gene bank EU372006.1)	

The amplification was carried out at the respective annealing temperature in 50 µl total reaction volume by using an RT-PCR kit (Sigma, USA) as per the manufacturer's protocol. Reagents were taken in a 0.2 ml thin-walled PCR tube. The PCR reaction consisted of 5µl of 10X PCR buffer, 3 µl of 25 mM $MgCl_2$, 1 µl of each Deoxynucleotide, RNase inhibitor (5U/ µl), eAMV-RT (5U/ µl), Fwd and Rev Primers (40 pmol./µl), AccuTaq LA DNA polymerase (10U/ µl), 31 µl Nuclease free water and 5 µl of CHIKV RNA (20 ng/ µl).

Table 4.2: Thermal cycle of the One-step Reverse Transcription Polymerase chain reaction

Temp.	Time	No. of cycles	Remarks
48^{0}C	45 min	1	Reverse transcription
95^{0}C	5 min	1	Initial denaturation
94^{0}C	45 sec	40	Denaturation
63^{0}C	45 sec		Primer annealing
72^{0}C	2 min		Primer extension
72^{0}C	10 min	1	Final extension
4^{0}C	Infinite	-	Hold

Transmission Electron Microscopy (TEM)

The purified Chikungunya virions were fixed in 4% formaldehyde (made in PBS), negatively stained with 1.5% phosphotungstic acid (PTA), pH 7.2 as described previously (Palmer et.al., 1988) with few modifications. Briefly, we placed 1.0 µl of the virus sample onto a carbon-coated Formvar-filmed copper grid (TAAB, UK) and allowed the purified Chikungunya virions to attach to the surface for one minute. The grids were washed three times in sterile triple distilled water by floating the grid on water droplets for 30 seconds each to remove sucrose and excess samples. Finally, the virions were negatively stained by floating the grid on a droplet of 1.5% PTA solution. The grid was dried on Whatman filter paper and was examined using a Transmission electron microscope (FEI Tecnai, Japan) operated at 75 kV at All India Institute of Medical Sciences, New Delhi.

CLONING OF CHIKV POLYPROTEIN GENE OF CHIKUNGUNYA VIRUS IN T/A CLONING VECTOR

Gene coding for ORF of structural Polyprotein of Chikungunya virus was cloned as left and right fragments in pTZ57R/T T/A cloning vector that was commercially available with Topo cloning kit (Fermentas, USA).

Bioinformatics Software

BioEdit and DNA star software were used for CHIKV polyprotein gene sequence analysis that included sequence similarity analysis, designing of primers, identification of reading frames and finding the internal restriction sites.

Oligonucleotide Primers Designing

CHIKV polyprotein gene-specific oligonucleotide primers used in the present study were newly designed based on the gene sequences of DRDE07 (NCBI Genbank accession no: EU372006) with the help of DNAstar software. The Oligonucleotide sequences were synthesized by MWG, Germany. Initially, a stock solution of 1000 p.mol/µl was prepared by adding the required volume of TE buffer. The working concentration of the primers (20pmol/µl) from original stocks was subsequently made in filtered Milli Q water and was used for PCR amplifications.

The nucleotide sequence of the CHIKV-specific primer pair and the characteristics of the amplicon are shown in Table 3.3.

Table 4.3: Primer sequences and the characteristics of CHIKV polyprotein-specific amplicon

Primer	**Sequences (5 '- 3')**	**Targeted region**	**Restriction Enzyme sites**	**Annealing Temp. (°C)**
CHIKYVLP Fwd **CHIKYVLP Rev**	TATACGTAATG GAG TTC ATC CCA ACC C TA CCTAGGTTA TTA TTC TTA GTG CCT GCT G	Full Poly-protein gene 3747 bp	*SnaB*I *Avr*II	58
CHIKYVLP Fwd **CHIKVLP MRev**	TATACGTAATG GAG TTC ATC CCA ACC C CAC GTG ACC TCG AGC CCT TCA	Left frag-ment 1952 bp	*SnaB*I *Xho*I (Natural site)	63
CHIKVLP MFwd **CHIKYVLP Rev**	TGA AGG GCT CGA GGT CAC GTG TA CCTAGGTTA TTA TTC TTA GTG CCT GCT G	Right fragment 1795 bp	*Xho*I (Natural site) *Avr*II	63

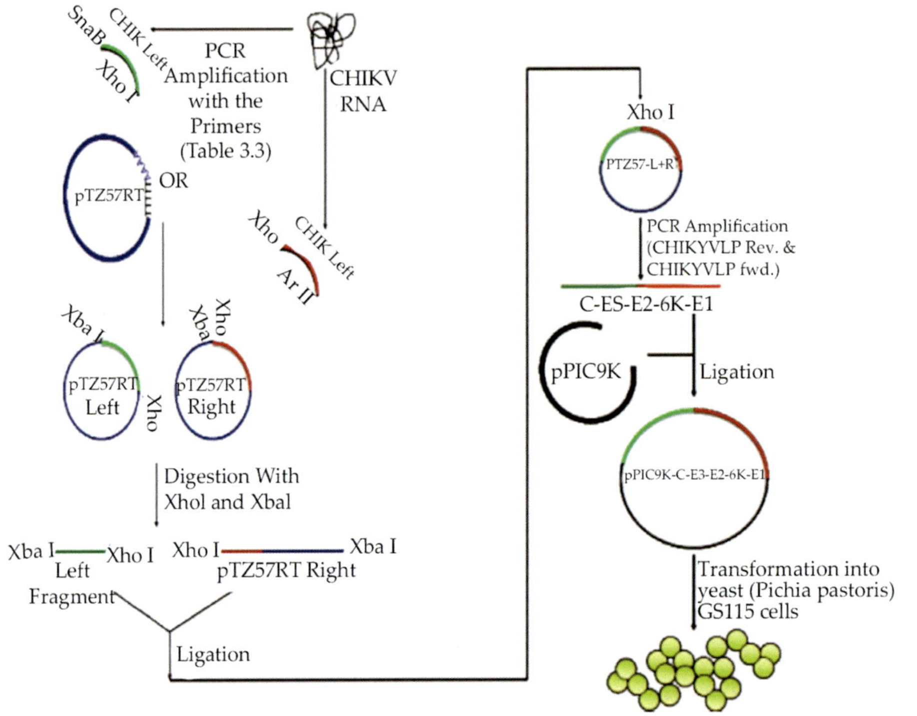

Figure 4.1: Schematic representation of cloning of structural polyprotein gene of Chikungunya virus into yeast *Pichia pastoris*.

Amplification of CHIKV Polyprotein Gene by one-step RT-PCR

The gene encoding CHIKV polyprotein was amplified as two fragments known as left and right fragments having a *XhoI* natural restriction site.

The conventional RT-PCR was performed with the above-mentioned primer sets targeting left and right fragments of the CHIKV polyprotein gene. The amplification was carried out in 50 µl total reaction volume by using an RT-PCR kit (Sigma, USA) as per the manufacturer's protocol. Reagents were taken in a 0.2 ml thin-walled PCR tube. The PCR reaction consisted of 5µl of 10X PCR buffer, 3 µl of 25 mM $MgCl_2$, 1 µl of each Deoxynucleotide, RNase inhibitor (5U/ µl), eAMV-RT (5U/ µl), Fwd and Rev Primers (40 pmol./µl), AccuTaq LA DNA polymerase (10U/ µl), 31 µl Nuclease free water and 5 µl of CHIKV RNA (20 ng/ µl).

Table 4.4: Thermal cycle of the One-step Reverse Transcription-Polymerase chain reaction for left and right fragments

Temp.	Time	No. of cycles	Remarks
48^0C	45 min	1	Reverse transcription
95^0C	5 min	1	Initial denaturation
94^0C	45 sec	40	Denaturation
63^0C	45 sec		Primer annealing
72^0C	2 min		Primer extension
72^0C	10 min	1	Final extension
4^0C	Infinite	-	Hold

Analysis of Amplified PCR Product with Agarose Gel Electrophoresis

The size and quantity of the PCR amplicon were confirmed by running it electrophoretically on 1% agarose gel as described by Sambrook et al., 1989. Briefly, 1% Agarose gel containing 0.5 µg/ml of ethidium bromide was made in 1X TAE buffer. Amplified product (10 ml) was mixed with 2 ¼l of 6X Gel loading dye and loaded along with a known molecular weight marker (1000bp DNA ladder) in an adjacent well. Electrophoresis was carried out at 5 volts/cm^2 until the tracking dye (Bromo phenol blue) passed out of the gel. Further, the amplicons were visualized in a Gel Documentation system (Bio-Rad, USA).

Purification of PCR Products

Amplified PCR product was purified by using the QIA quick PCR clean up kit (Qiagen, Germany) as per the manufacturer's protocol.

To the PCR product, 5 volumes of Buffer PB1 were added and mixed gently by vortexing. The mixture was transferred to the QIA quick spin column and centrifuged at 13000 rpm for 1 min at 4^0C. The flow-through was discarded and the column was washed with 0.75ml of buffer PE by centrifuging at 12000 rpm for 1 min at 4^0C. After discarding the flow-through, the column was given a dry spin at 13000 rpm for 1 min at 4^0C.

The column was placed in a fresh sterile microcentrifuge tube and DNA was eluted by adding 50μl EB buffer to the center of the QIA quick membrane and incubated for 5 min. The column was centrifuged at 13000 rpm for 1 min at 4^0C and the purified PCR product was stored at -20^0C until further use.

Ligation of Left and Right Fragments with pTZ57 Vector

Subsequently, ligation was performed at 16^0C overnight with 20 μl reaction volume using vector and purified PCR product by T4 DNA ligase enzyme. The purified PCR products (Left 1952 bp and Right 1795 bp) of the CHIKV polyprotein gene were separately ligated into pTZ57vector as follows:

5X T4 DNA ligase Buffer - 2 μl

pTZ57vector - 1 μl (100 ng)

Purified PCR products - 3 μl (300 ng) T4 DNA Ligase enzyme (10U) - 1 μl

Nuclease-free water - 13 μl

The ligated product was transformed into *E. coli* DH5α competent cells. Positive clones were selected by colony lysis screening and confirmed by restriction and PCR analysis.

Competent Cells Preparation

To clone the desired genes, the *E. coli* DH5α cells were made competent for transformation by treating with $CaCl_2$ as described by Sambrook et al., (1989). The protocol is as follows: 10 ml of LB broth was inoculated with a single colony from the plate and incubated on a shaker incubator at 150 rpm, 37^0C for 16 hrs. From this overnight culture, 1 ml was inoculated into 100 ml LB broth and incubated at 37^0C with shaking until the culture reached an O.D. of 0.4 to 0.6 at 600 nm (3-4 hrs incubation). The freshly grown culture was harvested at the log phase of growth by centrifugation at 4000 rpm for 10 min at 4^0C. The supernatant was discarded under the hood and the cell pellet was then resuspended in 20 ml of 100 mM ice-cold solution of $CaCl_2$ and kept on ice for 45 min. The cells were recovered by centrifuging as above and finally, the pellet was resuspended in 10 ml of 100 mM ice-cold $CaCl_2$ by gentle tapping, and centrifuging at 4000 rpm for 10 min at 4^0C. The supernatant was discarded and the cell pellet was resuspended in 2ml ice-cold 0.1M $CaCl_2$, and 1 ml of ice-cold 50% V/V glycerol. The cell suspension was gently mixed and aliquoted (100µl each) in pre-chilled sterile 1.5 ml microfuge tubes and stored at -80°C for further use.

Transformation

Hence prepared bacterial competent cells were transformed with the ligated constructs as described below-

An aliquot of frozen competent cells was thawed on ice. 10 µl of the ligated product was added to one aliquot of the competent cells along with one negative control. To the negative tube, only linearized pTZ57 plasmid was added. These samples were incubated on ice for 30 min. Heat shock was given to the cells in a water bath at 42°C for 90 sec and snap cooled on ice and kept for 5 min. Then, 1000 µl of LB Broth was added to each tube and incubated in a shaker at 37°C for 1 hr. The cells were finally centrifuged at 4000 rpm for 5 min and the pellet was resuspended in 100 µl of fresh LB broth and plated on LB agar having 100 µg/ml ampicillin, and incubated at 37°C overnight. The plates were incubated for 16 hrs at 37°C. Then the positive clones were confirmed by colony lysis screening and PCR analysis.

Screening of Recombinant Clones

After overnight incubation, the appeared colonies on the selection plate were counted. For the selection of the recombinant transformants, individual colonies were streaked on fresh LB agar plates having 50µg/ml ampicillin and incubated at 37°C overnight. Screening of recombinant pTZ57 left and pTZ57 right clones was carried out by the colony lysis method and confirmed by polymerase chain reaction as described below.

Colony Lysis of Transformants

The clones carrying plasmids with or without insert DNA were screened from individual colonies through the colony lysis method as described below.

For this, colonies obtained after transformation were streaked on LB agar plates having 50 µg/ml Ampicillin and incubated overnight at 37°C. Transformants from plates were picked and mixed thoroughly with 80 µl colony lysis buffer (100mM Tris HCl pH 8, 10mM EDTA, 10 mg/ml Lysozyme and 1 mg/ml RNase), incubated for 60 min at 37°C. An equal volume of phenol: chloroform (1:1v/v) was added to the mixture and vortexed. The lysate was centrifuged at 10000 rpm for 30 min at 4°C. Fifty microliters from the aqueous layer were mixed with 6X loading dye and analyzed by 1% agarose gel electrophoresis. The colonies running higher than the control plasmid were assumed as positive clones. These clones were further confirmed by polymerase chain reaction.

PCR Analysis of Positive Clones

PCR analysis of positive clones was done using the primers described previously. Correct integration would result in the amplification of 1.96 Kbp and 1.79 Kbp PCR products. PCR products were analyzed through 1% agarose gel along with a standard molecular weight marker.

Construction of pTZ57-C-E3-E2-6K-E1 Construct in DH5α Cells

Digestion of pTZ57Left and pTZ57 Right Construct

The pTZ57 Left and pTZ57 Right construct was digested with *XbaI* & *XhoI* restriction enzymes (Fermentas, USA) using digestion buffer supplied along with the enzymes. About 10µg of each DNA was subjected to double digestion in the presence of 5 units of each enzyme in the total volume of 100µl at 37^0C for 5 hrs. The enzymes were inactivated by incubating the mixtures at 65^0C for 10 min. The digested samples were run on 1% agarose gel along with a 1kb DNA marker. Digestion resulted in 1.9 Kbp release from the pTZ57 Left construct and 4.7 Kbp linearized pTZ57 Right construct.

Gel Purification of Digested Left Release and Right Constructs

Following restriction digestion, DNA was further purified *via* QIA quick Gel extraction kit (Qiagen, USA). The digested products were separated on 1% agarose gel in order to separate partial or undigested DNA from the digested linear DNA. The band that corresponds to the 1.9 Kbp left fragment and 4.0 Kbp linearized vector DNA were separately excised from the gel using a sterile sharp blade and kept in a separate microcentrifuge tube for calculating their weights. For gel purification, the following procedure were followed-

The agarose gel, containing the specific DNA band was excised with a clean, sharp scalpel. The gel slice was weighed and 3 volumes of buffer QG was added to 1 volume of gel. It was incubated at 50^0C for 10 min with vortexing in between. Then isopropanol was added to the sample in an equal volume to the original gel and was mixed thoroughly. The sample was then applied to the QIAquick spin column and centrifuged at 10000 rpm for 1 min. The flow-through was discarded and the column was placed in the same collection tube. 500 μl of buffer QG was added to the column and centrifuged at 10000 rpm for 1 min. The column was washed with 750 μl of buffer PE by centrifugation at 10000 rpm for 1 min. The column was placed in a new collection tube and again centrifuged at 10000 rpm for an additional 1 min to remove trace of wash buffer, if any. Next, the column was placed in a clean 1.5 ml Eppendorf tube and the DNA was eluted by adding 30 μl of nuclease-free water to the column, and centrifuging at 10000 rpm for 2 min. The collected purified amplicons were stored at -20^{0}C till use.

Ligation of Left Release and Linearized pTZ57 Right veCtor

Subsequently, ligation was performed at 16^{0}C overnight with 20 μl reaction volume using purified vector and insert by T4 DNA ligase enzyme. The purified insert (1952 bp) of the CHIKV polyprotein gene was separately ligated into the linearized pTZ57 Right vector as follows:

5X T4 DNA ligase Buffer - 2 μl

pTZ57 Right vector - 1 μl (100 ng)

Purified Insert - 3 μl (300 ng) T4 DNA Ligase enzyme (10U) - 1 μl

Nuclease-free water - 13 μl

The ligated product was transformed in *E. coli* DH5α competent cells by the heat shock method described as previously. Positive clones were selected by colony lysis screening and confirmed by restriction analysis.

Colony Lysis of Transformants

The clones carrying a plasmid with or without insert DNA were screened from individual colonies through the colony lysis method as described previously.

Restriction Digestion Analysis of Positive Clones

Plasmid DNA of some positive clones was isolated using QIAprep spin miniprep kit as described below and subjected to restriction digestion with *Xba* I enzymes. After digestion samples were electrophoresed through 1% agarose gel along with a standard molecular weight marker and visualized under UV illumination.

SUB CLONING OF CHIKV POLYPROTEIN GENE INTO PPIC9K YEAST TRANSFER VECTOR

The full CHIKV polyprotein gene was cloned in the pTZ57 vector. For constructing the pPIC9K-CHIKV-C-E3-E2-6K-E1 transfer vector, the full structural polyprotein Chikungunya virus was amplified from the pTZ57-C-E3-E2-6K-E1 construct by using CHIKYVLP forward and CHIKYVLP reverse primers. Briefly, the full-length CHIKV structural polyprotein gene was PCR amplified from the pTZ57-C-E3-E2-6K-E1 construct using high-fidelity *Pfu* polymerase (Fermentas, USA). The PCR reaction consisted of 5μl of 10X PCR buffer, 1.5mM $MgCl_{2,}$ 0.1mM of each dNTPs (dATP, dGTP, dCTP, dTTP), 20 p.mol. of each primer (CHIKYVLP FWD and CHIKYVLP REV), 1 unit of *Pfu* DNA polymerase and 1μl of template DNA. The total volume of the reaction mixture was made up to 50μl with nuclease-free water. The PCR reaction was performed in a gradient thermal cycler (Bio-Rad, Germany). The PCR conditions optimized are mentioned in Table 3.5 below.

Table 4.4: The PCR conditions optimized for amplification of the CHIKV structural polyprotein gene

Temp.	Time	No. of cycles	Remarks
48^0C	45 min	1	Reverse transcription
95^0C	5 min	1	Initial denaturation
94^0C	45 sec	40	Denaturation
58^0C	45 sec		Primer annealing
72^0C	3.30 min		Primer extension
72^0C	10 min	1	Final extension
4^0C	Infinite	-	Hold

PCR products were analyzed through 1% agarose gel along with a standard molecular weight marker.

Gel Purification of Full Structural Polyprotein Gene

The amplified product was purified using the QIA quick gel extraction kit (Qiagen, Germany), according to the manufacturer's protocol as described previously.

Plasmid Isolation (Purification of pPIC9K Yeast Transfer Plasmid DNA)

Cloning of full-length CHIKV Polyprotein gene was carried out in pPIC9K yeast transfer vector. The vector was purified from overnight grown culture using QIAprep spin miniprep kit (Qiagen, Germany), as per manufacturer's instructions given below: Transformed DH5α cells known to carry pPIC9K vector were incubated for 16-18 hrs at 37⁰C in LB broth having 100μg/ml Ampicillin. Five milliliters of overnight grown bacterial culture was pelleted by centrifugation at 10000 rpm for 3 min at room temperature. The bacterial cells were resuspended in 250μl resuspension buffer P1 having RNAse and Lyse Blue. 250μl lysis buffer P2 was added and mixed by inverting the tube 4-6 times or until the solution turns completely blue. 350μl neutralization buffer N3 was added and mixed immediately by inverting the tube 4-6 times until the solution turns colorless and centrifuged at 12000 rpm for 10 min at 4⁰C. The supernatant was applied onto the QIAprep spin column and centrifuged at 10000 rpm for 1 min at 4⁰C. The flow-through was discarded and the column was washed with 500μl binding buffer PB by centrifuged at 10000 rpm for 1 min at 4⁰C. The column was washed by adding 750μl wash buffer PE and centrifuged at 10000 rpm for 1 min at 4⁰C. A dry spin was given to the column for removing the residual wash buffer by centrifuging it at 10000 rpm for 2 min. The QIAprep spin column was placed in a clean 1.5 ml microcentrifuge tube. DNA was eluted in 50μl elution buffer EB by centrifuging for 2 min at 12000 rpm at 4⁰C. The plasmid DNA was stored at -20⁰C until used further.

Restriction Digestion of Purified PCR Product and the Plasmid DNA

Both purified PCR product and purified plasmid DNA were digested with *AvrII* and *SnaB*I restriction enzymes (Fermentas, USA) using digestion buffer supplied along with the enzymes. About 10μg of each DNA was subjected to double digestion in the presence of 5 units of each enzyme in the total volume of 100μl at 37⁰C for 5 hrs. The enzymes were inactivated by incubating the mixtures at 65⁰C for 10 min. The digested samples were run on 1% agarose gel along with a 1kb DNA marker.

Gel Purification of Digested Vector

Following restriction digestion of vector, the DNA products were further purified *via* QIAquick Gel extraction kit (Qiagen, USA). The digested products were separated on 1% agarose gel in order to separate partial or undigested DNA from the digested linear DNA. The band that corresponds to the linearized vector DNA was separately excised from the gel using a sterile sharp blade and kept in a separate microcentrifuge tube for calculating their weights. Gel extraction was carried out by the Quigen gel extraction kit described as above.

LIGATION OF PURIFIED CHIKV FULL-LENGTH POLYPROTEIN FRAGMENT WITH PPIC9K YEAST TRANSFER VECTOR

After digestion with *AvrII* and *SnaB*I restriction enzymes, digested insert and vector DNA were quantified using a Nanodrop spectrophotometer (Thermo Scientific, USA). To set up the ligation reaction, a 1:3 molar ratio of vector/insert was used based on the following formula.

ng of vector x Kb size of insert x Molar ratio of insert/vector = ng of insert size of vector in kb

The ligation mixture consisted of 10X T4 DNA ligase buffer, 1:3 ratio of vector/ insert, Nuclease free water and 5U/ml T4 DNA ligase enzyme (Fermentas, USA). Ligation was set up at 16^{0}C overnight in the thermal cycler, then ligase was inactivated by incubating at 65^{0}C for 10 min and stored at -20^{0}C until used for transformation experiment. The linearized pPIC9K plasmid DNA without insert was also ligated in a separate reaction to serve as a negative control.

Transformation of pPIC9K-CHIKV-C-E3-E2-6K-E1 Construct into Chemically Competent DH5α Cells

The pPIC9K-CHIKV-C-E3-E2-6K-E1 DNA was transformed into *E.coli* DH5α strain (Invitrogen, USA) *via the* heat shock method described earlier. For negative control linearized pPICK9K vector was also included in a separate transformation experiment.

Screening of Recombinant Clones

After overnight incubation, colonies that appeared on the selection plate were counted. For the selection of the recombinant transformants, individual colonies were streaked on fresh LB agar plates having 50μg/ml ampicillin and incubated at 37^{0}C overnight. Screening of recombinant pPIC9K-

CHIKV-C-E3-E2-6K-E1 clones was carried out by colony lysis method, restriction digestion, polymerase chain reaction and sequencing analysis.

Colony Lysis of Transformants

The clones carrying the plasmid with or without inset DNA were screened from individual colonies through the colony lysis method described earlier.

Restriction Digestion Analysis of Positive Clones

Plasmid DNA of some positive clones was isolated using QIAprep spin miniprep kit as described above and subjected to restriction digestion with *AvrII* and *SnaB*I enzymes along with pPIC9K plasmid DNA (without inset). After digestion samples were electrophoresed through 1% agarose gel along with a standard molecular weight marker and visualized under UV illumination.

PCR Analysis of Positive Clones

PCR analysis of positive clones was done using CHIKYVLP forward and CHIKYVLP Reverse primers. Correct integration would result in the amplification of a 3.74 Kbp PCR product.

Table 4.5: Thermal cycle of the Polymerase chain reaction for the full structural polyprotein gene

Temp.	Time	No. of cycles	Remarks
48^{0}C	45 min	1	Reverse transcription
95^{0}C	5 min	1	Initial denaturation
94^{0}C	45 sec	40	Denaturation
58^{0}C	45 sec		Primer annealing
72^{0}C	3.30 min		Primer extension
72^{0}C	10 min	1	Final extension
4^{0}C	Infinite	-	Hold

Sequencing Analysis of Positive Clones

The complete structural Polyprotein gene sequence was further confirmed through nucleotide sequencing using an ABI sequencer for any possible mutations introduced during the PCR step.

Cycle sequencing

Plasmid DNA sample that was positive through restriction digestion analysis and PCR was subjected to sequencing using ABI PRISM Big Dye® terminator v3.1cycle sequencing ready reaction kit (Applied Biosystems, USA). Plasmid DNA was sequenced both from the 3' end and 5' end using CHIKYVLP gene-specific primers and alpha-factor forward primer respectively. Briefly, a sequencing reaction was carried out in a final volume of 10 µl by mixing the Big Dye terminator mix containing the thermostable AmpliTaq DNA polymerase, dNTPs and four dye-labeled dideoxy nucleotide terminators (ddNTPs) and 25 ng of purified plasmid DNA, and either upstream or downstream primer in a PCR tube.

The reaction mixture was prepared in a 0.2 ml PCR.

- Nuclease-free water : 4 µl
- 5X big Dye Master Mix : 4 µl
- Sequencing Primer (3.2 pmol/µl) : 1 µl
- Purified plasmid DNA : 1 µl

Table 4.6: Thermal cycle for nucleotide sequencing of amplicons

Temperature	**Time**	**No. of cycles**	**Remarks**
96^0C	1 min	1	Initial denaturation
96^0C	10 sec	25	Denaturation
55^0C	5 sec		Primer annealing
60^0C	4 min		Primer extension/ chain termination
4^0C	Infinite	-	Hold

Purification of Sequencing Products by Centri-sep column

The purification of sequencing products was carried out to remove unincorporated dye terminators, employing the centri-sep protocol, as described below The centriSep columns were initially tapped to settle the gel at the bottom. The top cap was removed and 800 ml of autoclaved MQ water was applied. The columns were then allowed to stand for 30 min at RT. Columns were inverted and vortexed for proper hydration of gel. All air bubbles were removed by tapping the column. Then gel was allowed to settle by keeping the column stand on a rack. The top column cap and end stopper were removed and Columns were placed on wash tubes. Then columns were centrifuged at 8000xg for 5 min to remove all water contents. The columns were placed onto a 1.5 ml Eppendorf tube and samples were added at the center of the column and then centrifuged at 8000xg for 5 min. Thus obtained purified sample was vacuum dried. 15 ml of Hi-di formamide was added to the dried sample, and mixed properly by vortexing and centrifuging. The products were then denatured at 95^{0}C for 5 min, 4^{0}C for 7 min and then loaded into ABI PRISM™ 3130 Genetic Analyzer (Applied Biosystems, USA) for nucleotide sequencing.

Sequence analysis

Sequencing data obtained were subjected to BLAST at http://www.ncbi.nlm.nih.gov/BLAST, to find the closest possible match from available sequences in GenBank and further analyzed for reading frame and orientation of the insert using DNA star software.

TRANSFORMATION OF THE PPIC9K-CHIKV-C-E3-E2-6K-E1 RECOMBINANT CONSTRUCT INTO YEAST (*PICHIA PASTORIS*) GS115 STRAIN

Preparation of Electro-competent Yeast Cells

A single colony of GS115 from the YPD agar plate was inoculated into 5ml YPD broth and was incubated at 30^{0}C for 16hrs with shaking (250-280rpm). This overnight grown culture (0.5ml) was inoculated into 500ml fresh YPD broth in a 2L flask and allowed to grow at 28^{0}C to reach an A_{600} reached 1.3 to 1.5. The cells were pelleted at 4000 rpm for 5min at 4^{0}C and suspended in 500ml ice-cold sterile distilled water. The cells were repelletized as above and were resuspended in 250ml sterile ice-cold distilled water. The cells were again pelleted at 4^{0}C as above and finally resuspended in 20 ml sterile ice-cold 1M sorbitol. The cells were again pelleted and the cell pellets were resuspended finally in 1.5ml of sterile ice-cold 1M sorbitol and aliquoted as 80µl in sterile ice-cold 1.5ml micro centrifuging tubes and used immediately.

Linearization of the pPIC9K-CHIKV-C-E3-E2-6K-E1 Construct

Recombinant plasmid pPIC9K-CHIKV-C-E3-E2-6K-E1 carrying full structural polyprotein gene was isolated from 25ml overnight grown recombinant bacterial culture by using QIAprep spin miniprep kit (Qiagen, USA) as described earlier. The recombinant plasmid DNA (~20µg) was linearized by digesting with *Sac I* enzyme to integrate the transgene at the His4 locus on the *Pichia* genome and also to generate HIS $^{+}$ Mut^{+} transformants in *Pichia pastoris* GS115 cells. The restriction digestion was carried out for 6 hrs as previously described.

PURIFICATION OF THE LINEARIZED PPIC9K-CHIKV-C-E3-E2-6K-E1 CONSTRUCT

After digestion, the DNA was purified using the QIAquick Gel extraction kit as described above. After purification, concentrations of the DNA samples were measured and stored at -20^{0}C until used for transformation. Linearization of pPICK9K DNA with or without insert at *Sac I* site results in homologous recombination within the HIS4 gene of the yeast genome while electroporation and hence Mut^{+} recombinants will be generated.

Yeast Transformation by Electroporation

Ten micrograms of the linear DNA were used to transform fresh electrocompetent *P. pastoris* cells *via* electroporation using Bio-Rad Gene Pulsar Xcell™ electroporation system (Bio-Rad Laboratories, USA) at three different voltages to optimize the electroporation conditions. Briefly, freshly prepared competent cells (80µl) were mixed with 10µg each of linearized plasmid, and transferred to a pre-cooled sterile electroporation cuvette (0.2 cm) (Eppendorf, Germany). After incubating the cells for 30 minutes on ice, the cuvette was placed into the cuvette holder in the electroporator and three different voltages (1600V, 1800V and 2000V) 20µF capacitance and 200Ω resistance were applied individually to each cuvette immediately with default time settings (2 seconds). Immediately after the electric pulse (within 8 ms), one milliliter of ice-cold 1M sorbitol was added to the cuvette and the contents were transferred to a sterile microfuge tube and incubated at 200rpm, 28^{0}C for 2 hrs in the shaker at 180 rpm. After incubation DNA cell mixture was centrifuged at 1500g for 5 min at 28^{0}C and resuspended in 200µl YPD and this cell suspension was plated on SD-His plates and incubated at 28^{0}C for 2 days. The parent pPIC9K without insert, linearized with *Sac I* was also transformed similarly for negative control.

SCREENING OF POSITIVE TRANSFORMANTS (*PICHIA* CLONE) BY GENETICIN SENSITIVITY ASSAY AND PCR

Pichia transformants were screened through Geneticin (G418) sensitivity assay, PCR and qRT-PCR analysis to select the colonies with inserted target DNA.

Geneticin (G418) Sensitivity Assay

After transformation colonies obtained on SD agar plates was screened for different concentration of Geneticin. Three hundred and sixty-five transformed colonies bearing the chromosomally integrated copies of the pPIC9K-CHIKV-C-E3-E2-6K-E1 were screened for single, double or multiple copy integrants through replica plating on YPD plates containing different concentrations of Geneticin (250µg, 500µg and 750µg). Plates were incubated at 28^{0}C for 72 hrs. The growth obtained was scored with plus (+) and minus (-) for the presence or absence of growth respectively on the selection plate. To further confirm the transformants PCR was performed from the genomic DNA isolated from selected colonies.

Isolation of Genomic DNA from Yeast Transformants

A total of twenty clones were randomly picked up from all the three categories (3, 6 and 11 clones each from 250 µg/ml, 500 µg/ml and 750 µg/ml plates respectively) and were inoculated into 10 ml of YPD broth and grown at 28°C until the A_{600} reached 2-3 (16-18 hrs of incubation).

2 ml culture was taken and harvested by centrifugation at 1500g for 10 min at room temperature and washed once with 5 ml sterile water by centrifuging at 1500 g for 10 min at R.T. Parent host cells (GS115-untransformed) that were grown in a similar way were used as control. Again cell pellet was washed with sterile water twice and the cells were resuspended in 2ml of freshly prepared SCED buffer. After thorough mixing, the tubes were sonicated for 2 min by using an ultra sonicator to achieve 80% spheroplasting. 400 µl of 1% SDS was added, mixed gently and kept on ice for 5 min. The cell debris was precipitated by adding 1.5ml of 5M Potassium acetate (pH 8.9) and centrifugation at 10000 rpm for 10min at 4^{0}C.

Supernatant from the above step was taken in a new tube and an equal volume of phenol: chloroform was added and centrifuged at 10000 rpm for 10min at 4^{0}C. The aqueous phase was split into two microfuge tubes and

DNA was precipitated by adding 0.5 volume of 7.5 M ammonium acetate (pH 5.0) and two volumes of ethanol. The tubes were placed at -80^{0}C for 30 min and DNA was pelleted by centrifuging at 14,000 g for 20 min at 4^{0}C. Pellets were washed once with 1 ml of 70% ethyl alcohol at 10000 rpm for 10 min and air-dried. All DNA samples were finally suspended in 50 µl of TE (pH 7.4). 5µl of the above DNA was run on 1 % Agarose gel to assess the quality of purified DNA and the remaining DNA was stored at -20^{0}C for further use.

Analysis by PCR

For preliminary screening of recombinant clones having differential copy numbers of the transgene, a simple PCR was performed using equal concentrations of genomic DNA. A total of 20 clones showing resistance to different concentrations of Geneticin viz, 0.25, 0.5 and 0.75 mg/ml were randomly selected and subjected to genomic DNA PCR using AOX1 forward and CHIKYVLP reverse primers as described previously.

Table 4.6: Primer sequence and characteristics of CHIKV polyprotein amplicon

Primer	Sequences (5 '- 3')	Targeted region	Annealing Temp. (^{0}C)
AOX Fwd **CHIKYVLP Rev**	TAC TAT TGC CAG CAT TGC TGC TA CCTAGGTTA TTA TTC TTA GTG CCT GCT G	Full Polyprotein gene with AOX promoter region 3947 bp	58

PCR analysis of positive clones was done using AOX forward and CHIKYVLP reverse primers. Correct integration would result in the amplification of a 3.94 kbp PCR product.

Table 4.7: Thermal cycle of the Polymerase chain reaction for the full structural polyprotein gene

Temp.	Time	No. of cycles	Remarks
48^{0}C	45 min	1	Reverse transcription
95^{0}C	5 min	1	Initial denaturation
94^{0}C	45 sec	35	Denaturation
58^{0}C	45 sec		Primer annealing
72^{0}C	4 min		Primer extension

72^{0}C	10 min	1	Final extension
4^{0}C	Infinite	-	Hold

Optimization of Recombinant Protein Expression

Finally, PCR-positive His^+ Mut^+ *Pichia* clones were selected for induction. The optimal method and growth conditions necessary for the expression of the target protein were standardized. The expression conditions viz methanol concentration (0.5-2.5%), type of medium (YPGy or BMGM), pH of the medium (6 - 8.5) and the time of harvest (24 h, 48 h, 72 h and 96 h) were tested in order to get the intact CHIK-VLPs expressed in abundance without any host-specific proteolytic cleavage.

Methanol Optimization of Transformants

Induction of protein expression was done as described previously (Cregg et al., 1987) with some modifications. PCR positive His^+ Mut^+ *Pichia* clones were selected for methanol induction. The glycerol stock of the above *Pichia* clone was inoculated into 50 ml of YPGy containing 500 μg/mL Geneticin along with negative control (*Pichia* transformed with pPICK9K without insert) and was incubated at 28^{0}C in a shaker incubator at 200 rpm until the culture reached an A_{600} of 4-5 for induction, the cells were harvested by centrifugation at 3,000 × g for 10 min at room temperature and the cell pellets were resuspended in a required volume of fresh YPM induction media as to get an A_{600} of 3 in all. Several methanol concentrations ranging from 0.5 to 2.5% (0.5%, 1%, 1.5%, 2% and 2.5%) were tried in order to choose the optimum concentration of methanol for induction in case of shake flask culture. Incubation was continued at 28^{0}C on an orbitary shaker (200 rpm) for four days. 2 ml culture was collected once every 24 hours and the required volume of methanol was added to every flask once every 24 hours to sustain induction. Supernatant collected both from pre-induced and induced cultures were concentrated through acetone precipitation and analyzed for the expression of CHIK-VLPs on discontinuous polyacrylamide gel electrophoresis under denaturing conditions.

MEDIA OPTIMIZATION OF CHIK-VLPS EXPRESSION IN THE *PICHIA* SYSTEM

PCR positive His^+ Mut^+ *Pichia* clone was selected for media optimization of expression. The glycerol stock of the above *Pichia* clone was inoculated into 50 ml of either YPGy or BMGM taken in a 500 ml conical flask along with negative control (*Pichia* transformed with pPICK9K without insert) and incubated at 28⁰C in a shaker incubator at 200 rpm until the culture reached an A_{600} of 4-5. The cells were harvested by centrifugation at 3,000 × g for 10 min at room temperature and the cell pellets were resuspended in the required volume of either fresh YPM induction media or BMM so as to get an A_{600} of 3 in all. Incubation was continued at 28⁰C on an orbitary shaker (200 rpm) for four days. To sustain induction, the required volume of methanol was added to every flask once every 24 hours. Culture supernatants were collected at different time points ranging from 16-96 h (24 h, 48 h, 72 h and 96 h) and were concentrated to 1/10 of their original volume using 10 kDa molecular weight cut off filters (Millipore Corporation, USA) by centrifuging at 4000 g for 30 min at 4⁰C. Protease inhibitor cocktail (Amersco, USA) was added to the concentrated samples and the samples were stored at -80⁰C until all the time points were collected. The final protein obtained after optimization of the expression conditions obtained from culture supernatants was determined through Bradford assay against BSA standards.

Protein Estimation of CHIK-VLPs

The amount of the protein produced by the clones was assayed by the dye-binding assay (Bradford, 1976). Aliquots of 10, 20, 40 and 60 μl of protein solutions from each sample was diluted to 100 μl with TE and to this 1ml of Bradford reagent (Appendix) was added and mixed. The A_{595} nm of the color development was read spectrophotometrically. The concentration was deduced from the standard curve drawn using BSA at different concentrations.

Detection and Confirmation of the CHIK-VLPs

Proteins expressed by *Pichia* clones carrying the Chikungunya polyprotein gene were detected by SDS-PAGE using a discontinuous buffer system as described earlier, followed by western blotting as per standard procedures (Sambrook et al., 1989). Clone without insert was used as a negative control.

Immunoblotting of Yeast-derived CHIK-VLPs

The selected fractions collected were electrophoresed on SDS-PAGE under reduced conditions as described earlier and separated proteins were blotted onto an Immobilon-P membrane (Millipore, India) using tris-glycine transfer buffer using semi-dry blotting apparatus (Bio-Rad-USA). The blot was blocked for 2 h in the blocking buffer. The target protein was reacted first with rabbit anti-CHIKV E2 antibodies (in-house) and then with anti-rabbit HRP conjugate. Finally, signals were developed using DAB-H_2O_2 substrate/chromogen solution.

Purification of the Yeast Derived CHIK-VLPs by Ultracentrifugation

The VLPs in the supernatant were purified by ultracentrifugation through a discontinuous sucrose gradient as described previously (Athmaram et al., 2013). Briefly, a discontinuous sucrose gradient was prepared by the layering of 60% and 20% (w/v) sucrose solution made in TNE buffer containing 50 mM Tris-HCl, pH 7.2, 1mM EDTA, 100 mM NaCl. Concentrated VLPs were layered over a discontinuous sucrose gradient and centrifuged in a TH-641 swinging bucket rotor (Thermo Scientific, USA) for 16 h at 32,000 rpm at 4^0C. The gradient fractions and 20-60% interface were harvested separately. The collected fractions were then analyzed by SDS-PAGE and western blot analysis for the presence of CHIKV structural polyprotein.

Characterization and Confirmation of Purified CHIK-VLPs

The purified CHIK-VLPs were characterized and confirmed by SDS-PAGE analysis, immunoblotting, ELISA and TEM as described earlier.

SDS-PAGE Analysis of Purified CHIK-VLPs

The fractions collected after ultracentrifugation were analyzed by 10% sodium dodecyl sulfate-polyacrylamide gel electrophoresis (SDS-PAGE) and visualized by Coomassie staining. The procedure followed was as described previously.

Western Blot Analysis of Purified CHIKV

The same fractions were also subjected to western blotting using rabbit polyclonal antibodies raised against recombinant Chikungunya E2 protein, mouse monoclonal antibodies raised against recombinant Chikungunya E1 protein and rabbit polyclonal antibodies raised against Chikungunya virus (obtained from the Division of Virology, DRDE, Gwalior) as described earlier.

Transmission Electron Microscopy (TEM)

The purified CHIK-VLPs were fixed in 4% formaldehyde (made in PBS) and negatively stained with 1.5% phosphotungstic acid (PTA), pH 7.2 as described previously (Palmer & Martin, 1988) with few modifications. Briefly, 1.0 μl of the VLPs were placed onto a carbon-coated Formvar-filmed copper grid (TAAB, UK) and allowed the CHIK-VLPs to attach to the surface for 1 min. The grid was washed thrice in sterile triple distilled water by floating the grid on water droplets for 45 seconds to remove excess sample and sucrose. Finally, the VLPs were negatively stained by 1.5% PTA solution *via* floating the grid droplet. The air-dried grid was examined using a Transmission electron microscope (FEI Tecnai, Japan) operated at 75 kV at Punjab University, Chandigarh.

Reactivity of CHIK-VLPs with Standard Anti-CHIKV Sera

The antigenicity of CHIK-VLPs was further confirmed using rabbit polyclonal serum raised against purified native CHIKV and recombinant E2-protein. The CHIK- VLPs used as antigen to coat microplates and their reactivity to anti-CHIKV native antigen sera and anti-CHIKV E2 specific serum was examined. Two-fold serial dilutions of rabbit serum starting from 1:00 dilution were subjected to the ELISA to detect antibodies. Maxisorp ninety-six-well plate (Nunc) was coated with CHIK-VLPs (300ng/well in coating buffer) and incubated at 4^{0}C overnight. The wells were blocked with 3% BSA in PBST (PBS having 0.05% tween-20) and the plate was incubated at 37^{0}C for 4 hours. The wells were washed five times with PBST.

In-house generated rabbit anti-E2 specific polyclonal antibodies and rabbit anti-CHIKV antibodies were added to each well and incubated at 37^{0}C for 1 hour. The plate was washed with PBST five times and subsequently reacted with goat anti-rabbit horse radish peroxidase conjugated IgG (Sigma, USA) (1:10000 dilution) and incubated at 37^{0}C for 1 hour. The wells were washed with PBST and color was developed using TMB/ H_2O_2 substrate chromogen (Sigma, USA) at room temperature. Following 5 minutes the reaction was stopped by adding 1 N H_2SO_4. Absorbance was recorded at 450nm by using a microplate reader (Biotek, USA).

EVALUATION OF CHIK-VLPS AS A DIAGNOSTIC INTERMEDIATE IN SEROLOGICAL DIAGNOSIS

Optimization of CHIK-VLPs for IgM ELISA

To determine the optimal concentration of yeast-derived CHIK-VLPs for detection of CHIKV IgM by indirect ELISA, the CHIK-VLPs were serially diluted from 10μg/ml to 1μg/ml. Confirmed positive and negative patient serum samples were then tested against different dilutions of CHIK-VLPs as the antigen. The highest ratio of absorbance value for positive to negative serum was obtained and was therefore used in further experiments to evaluate the diagnostic potential for detection of the CHIKV-specific IgM antibody.

Optimization of in-house IgM Microplate ELISA

An indirect microplate IgM ELISA was standardized using the purified CHIK- VLPs and recombinant E2 proteins. The purified proteins were diluted in 0.1M carbonate buffer, pH 9.6, and used for coating in a 96-well microtiter plate (300ng/well) and incubated at 37^{0}C for 2 h. The coated wells were washed once with 1× PBS and then blocked with 3% BSA in 1× PBS overnight at 4^{0}C. The following washing as above 100μl of CHIKV suspected patient sera at a dilution of 1:100 made in 1× PBS were added in the wells and incubated for 1h at 37^{0}C. The plate was incubated with anti-human IgM HRP conjugate (1:3000 dilutions in 3% BSA) followed by washing steps. The reaction was developed with 100μl of tetramethyl benzidine (TMB) substrate and kept at RT for 5 min. The peroxidase reaction was terminated with 100μl of 1 N H_2SO_4 and the absorbance was read at 450 nm in an ELISA reader.

COMPARATIVE EVALUATION OF CHIK-VLPS AND RE2 PROTEIN ANTIGEN-BASED IGM MICROPLATE ELISA WITH RESPECT TO NATIVE CHIKV-BASED IGM ELISA

The panel of 100 serum samples including 40 CHIKV suspected clinical samples, 20 each Dengue, JE infected patient sera samples and 20 healthy sera samples were processed for CHIKV detection by CHIK-VLP and rCHIK-E2 protein-based IgM ELISA. The specificity and sensitivity of the CHIK-VLP and rCHIK-E2 antigens were compared and evaluated keeping native antigen-based ELISA as a reference. All the samples were evaluated separately with the above proteins and the correlation, sensitivity, specificity, positive predictive value and negative predictive values were eventually calculated.

Determination of Cross-Reactivity

In order to determine cross-reactivity, panels of the sera positive for Dengue and Japanese encephalitis (20 for each) were used (Dash et al., 2006, 2007). Sera from apparently healthy individuals were taken as negative control and CHIKV patients' sera (N=20) were used as positive samples. All the samples were evaluated with the CHIK- VLPs, rCHIK-E2 and native antigens separately. The 96-wells of the microtiter plate were coated with 300 ng of antigen (native or recombinant) and allowed to react with the sera positive for Dengue, Japanese encephalitis, and Chikungunya. The reaction was further carried out as described before.

Endotoxin Estimation of the Purified CHIK-VLPs

The endotoxin level of the purified protein was measured by Limulus Amoebocyte Lysates (LAL) QCL-1000 kit (Cambrex Biosciences, USA) as per the manufacturer's protocol. Briefly, 25 μl of purified protein was diluted in an equal volume of LAL reagent water. From this diluted sample, 25 μl was applied to a PTS test cartridge (Lot No. 3420179, sensitivity range 5—0.05EU/mL.) and was analyzed for endotoxin concentration.

Evaluation of the Immunogenic Potential of CHIK-VLPs in BALB/c Mice

The immunogenicity of CHIK-VLPs as a vaccine candidate against CHIKV in Balb/c mice was evaluated in 4-5 week old female Balb/c mice. All the animals were immunized intradermally with different doses of CHIK-VLPs with Freund's adjuvant following standard immunization protocol. Both humoral and cell-mediated immune responses were evaluated. To determine humoral immune response, different techniques like ELISA, IgG Isotyping and PRNT were carried out. Induction of cell-mediated immune response was confirmed through cytokine production assay by ELISA.

For this study, forty healthy 4-week-old BALB/c mice were made into 4 groups each with ten animals. The animals were found to be sero negative for the Chikungunya virus. Groups 1, Group 2 and Group 3 were immunized intradermally each with 40μg, 20μg and 10μg of yeast-derived CHIK-VLPs in Freund's complete adjuvant (FCA) (Sigma, USA) and control animals (group 4) were immunized each with the PBS+ FCA. After two weeks, these animals were boosted once with the same amount of protein in combination with Freund's incomplete adjuvant (FIA) (Sigma, USA). Control animals were also boosted with PBS. To determine humoral and cell-mediated responses all groups were boosted with the same formulation on 14, and 28 days after the first immunization.

EVALUATION OF HUMORAL IMMUNE RESPONSE IMMUNIZATION SCHEDULE

The prime dose was given on day 0 followed by two boosters on days 14 and 28. Blood was collected from retro-orbital plexus with heparinized blood capillaries from each group on days: 0, 14, 28 42, 56 and 140 days after the first immunization. Sera were separated from all the samples and were stored at -80^{0}C until use.

S.N.	Group
1.	40 μg CHIK-VLPs
2.	20 μg CHIK-VLPs
3.	10 μg CHIK-VLPs
4.	Control

(A)

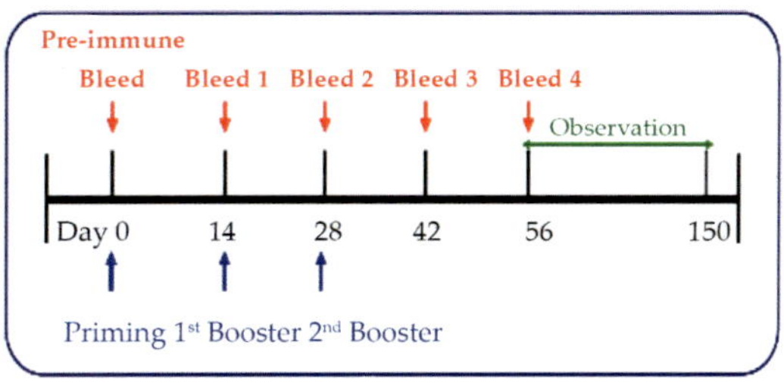

(B)

Figure 4.4: Immune responses and protective potential CHIK-VLPs were evaluated in a mouse model. (a) Balb/c mice (10/group) were immunized with different doses of CHIK- VLPs in formulation Freund's adjuvant. (b) Schematic representation of the immunization schedule.

Determination of Antibody Titer through ELISA

The anti-CHIK-VLPs IgG antibody response against CHIK-VLPs was determined on serum samples collected from individual mice at 14, 28, 42, 56 and 140 days post- vaccination. Sera were tested for anti-CHIK-VLPs antibody by standard indirect ELISA technique. Briefly, a 96-well microtiter plate (Nunc-Immuno Plate MaxiSorp) was coated with CHIK-VLPs as antigen at 300ng/well in coating buffer (pH 9.6), overnight at 4^{0}C, and the next day blocked with 3% BSA (Sigma, USA) in PBST for 4 hours at 37^{0}C. The wells were then washed five times with PBST, incubated with two-fold serial dilutions of the post-vaccinated sera starting with 1:250 to 1:51200 dilutions were incubated in triplicate wells (100µl/well) including healthy non-vaccinated sera prepared in PBST, for 1 h at 37^{0}C then washed five times with PBST. Bound antibodies were detected by HRP- labeled goat anti-mouse IgG (Sigma, USA) (working dilution 1:5,000) followed by washing and development with TMB/H_2O_2 (Sigma, USA) as substrate chromogen.

Finally, color development was stopped using 1N H_2SO_4 and the plate was read at 450 nm by a microplate reader (Biotek Instruments, Winooski, USA). The cut-off value for the assays was calculated as the mean absorbance (+2 SD) from sera of the control group assayed at 1:250 dilutions. The endpoint IgG titers were calculated as reciprocal of the highest serum dilution giving an absorbance more than the cut-off.

Similar indirect ELISA was performed for evaluating the potential of CHIK-VLPs in recognizing native CHIKV. In this, method 300 ng/well of purified native CHIKV was coated as antigen and the rest procedure remain the same.

Antibody Isotyping

The antibody profile of the post-vaccinated mice sera was determined through isotyping using a mouse antibody subtyping kit (Sigma, USA) following the manufacturer's protocol. Briefly, the antigen-coated ELISA plate was incubated with 1:1000 dilution (100µl) of immunized mice sera and incubated for 1 hr at 37^{0}C and then after washing thrice with PBST, wells were incubated with 1:1000 dilution (100µl) of goat anti-mouse IgG each subtype-specific antibodies (IgG1, IgG2a, IgG2b, IgG3) (Sigma, USA), separately and incubated at 37^{0}C for 1 h. After washing as above, 1:5000 dilution of rabbit anti-goat IgG HRP conjugate was applied and incubated at 37^{0}C for 30 min. Following washing with PBST, plates were developed using TMB/H_2O_2 as substrate chromogen and absorbance was measured at 450 nm using a microplate reader.

Immunofluorescence Assay

Sera samples were tested in an immunofluorescence assay for their ability to recognize the Chikungunya virus. Vero cells seeded on coverslip in a 6 well plate were used in this experiment. When cells attained 90% confluency, they were rinsed once with virus diluent (MEM without serum). Following washing, 10^3 PFU of Chikungunya virus was added to the respective test wells. The plates were incubated at 37^{0}C forl h, with shaking at 20 min intervals. Now, the cell monolayer was rinsed once with PBS and then MEM containing 2% FBS was added and incubated further at 37^{0}C for 24 hrs. The cells on coverslips were rinsed thrice with PBS and fixed with chilled methanol for 30 min. The cells were washed with PBS and blocked with 5% BSA for 2h at 37^{0}C. The cells were then washed thrice with PBS and incubated with PBS containing 0.1 % Triton X- 100 for 15 min to permeabilize the cells and washed with PBS. The cells were incubated for 1h at 37^{0}C with a 1:1000 dilution of hyperimmune sera raised against CHIK-VLPs. Similarly, dilution of pre-immune sera was used as the control. The cells were then washed thrice with PBS and then incubated with Fluorescein isothiocyanate (FITC) - conjugated goat anti-mouse antibody (1:100) (Sigma, USA) for 45 min at room temperature in dark. Cells were then washed and fluorescence was visualized using a Carl-Zeiss Aximot 2 (Olympus IX 71, Germany) microscope.

IN-VITRO NEUTRALIZATION ACTIVITY OF MICE SERA IMMUNIZED WITH CHIK-VLPS

In-vitro neutralization activity of mice sera immunized with CHIK–VLPs was carried out using two different techniques *viz* plaque reduction neutralization test (PRNT) and immunofluorescence assay (IFA). Sera samples were heat-inactivated at 56^{0}C for 30 minutes. Two-fold serial dilutions from 1:8 to 1:4196 were prepared in virus diluents (MEM with L-glutamine). Serially two-fold diluted serum was added to an equal volume of the CHIKV containing 10^2 pfu. The virus control of the experiment contained the CHIKV diluted in the virus diluent without serum. The serum/virus mixtures were incubated at 37^{0}C for one hour. This mixture was used to infect Vero cells for both PRNT and IFA. Vero cell monolayers, prepared in 24 well plates were infected with 200 µl/well of the serum/virus mixture.

Briefly in PRNT, Plates were incubated at 37^{0}C for one hour. The serum/virus mixtures were completely removed from the wells and the wells were overlaid with 1ml/well of MEM containing 2% FBS and 1.25% methyl cellulose (Sigma, USA). Plates were incubated at 37°C in 5% CO_2 for 3 days and the overlay media was removed after 3 days and cells were washed with PBS and fixed with chilled methanol for 1 hr. The fixed cell monolayers were stained with 0.25% crystal violet. The plaques formed were counted. The neutralizing titer is considered as the highest dilution of the sera that showed more than 50% reduction in plaque number, compared to virus control (serum negative control).

Whereas in IFA, following 24 hrs infection, immunofluorescence was developed by using anti-CHIKE2 and Fluorescein isothiocyanate (FITC) - conjugated goat anti-rabbit antibody (1:100) (Sigma, USA) as primary and secondary antibodies. Cells were then washed and fluorescence was visualized using a Carl-Zeiss Aximot 2 (Olympus IX 71, Germany) microscope. The highest dilution of sera that showed a reduction in fluorescence as compared to virus control was considered as the neutralization titer.

In Vivo Neutralization Test

In-vivo neutralization activity of mice sera, immunized with CHIK-VLPs was determined via passive immunization of purified IgG intraperitoneally as described previously (Cekinovic et al., 2008; Foo et al., 2007). Total IgG was purified from post- vaccinated sera (42 days post-immunization) by using a protein-A column (Sigma, USA). 10μg of purified IgG raised against yeast-derived CHIK-VLPs were immunized to suckling mice (2 days old, n=10) via the intraperitoneal route. For the control set, the same amount of non-specific IgG from pre-immune sera was used. After 48 hrs of IgG immunization, different groups of suckling mice were subcutaneously inoculated with 106 PFU of CHIKV. Symptoms were recorded at a regular interval of 24 h up to 10 days post- infection. Gain in body weight, percentage survival and serum viremia were determined. On days 3 and 6 after CHIKV inoculation, 3 mice pups in each experimental and control group were bled to determine serum viremia via real-time RT-PCR as described earlier (Agarwal et al., 2013).

A SYBR Green-I based Real Time RT-PCR

SYBR Green I based one-step real-time quantitative RT-PCR was performed using a primer pair: forward primer: CHIK1: 5’-ACGCAGTTGAGCGAAGCAC-3’ and reverse primer: CHIK2: 5’-CTGAAGACATTGGCCCCAC-3’ targeting to a highly conserved region of E1 gene of CHIKV (Dash et al., 2008). The quantitative RT-PCR was carried out using SS III Platinum one-step qRT-PCR kit (Invitrogen, Carlsbad, CA) in the Mx3000P system (Stratagene, La Jolla, CA). Samples were assayed in a 25 μL reaction volume containing 12.5 μL of 2X Master mix, 0.125 μL (0.25 μmol) each of forward and reverse primers, 0.25 μL of enzyme mix comprising Taq DNA polymerase and reverse transcriptase, 9.5

μL of nuclease-free water and 2.5 μL of RNA. The thermal profile consisted of 30 min of reverse transcription at 50^0C, 10 min of polymerase activation at 95^0C, followed by 40 cycles of PCR at 95^0C for 30s, 55^0C for 60s, and 72^0C for 30s. Following amplification, a melting curve analysis was performed with the melting curve analysis software of the Mx3000P according to the instructions of the manufacturer. Positive and negative template control was also included in all experiments.

Construction of standard curve and determination of detection limit

The standard curve was constructed to ascertain the detection limit of SYBR Green I based Real-time RT-PCR using CHIKV RNA. Briefly, Purified RNA was quantified by a Nanodrop spectrophotometer and 10-fold serial dilutions (10^{11}-10^0 RNA copies/ μL) were prepared and subjected to real-time RT-PCR. The Ct values obtained against the known concentration of serially diluted RNA were used for the construction of the standard curve. The quantity of RNA as determined by the Nanodrop spectrophotometer was converted to molecular copies, using the following formula, Y (molecules/ μL) = $[X(g/\mu L)/\{\text{transcript length(nucleotides)} \times 340\}] \times 6.023 \times 10^{23}$

Assessment of Cell-mediated Immune Response

Preparation of single cell suspension of splenocytes

On day 7 of post-booster vaccination, three mice from all the groups were randomly selected, sacrificed and their spleens were removed aseptically. Briefly, single cell suspension of splenocytes was prepared by maceration of spleens. The suspension was centrifuged at 2500 rpm for 8 min at 4^0C and the supernatant was discarded. Chilled lysis buffer (2ml) was added to the pellet and incubated on ice for 10 min. The volume of the samples was made up to 10 ml with RPMI incomplete media and centrifuged at 2500 rpm for 8 min at 4^0C. The supernatant was discarded and cells were incubated with 2 ml chilled lysis buffer for 5 min and centrifuged again. The supernatant was discarded and pellet was washed with RPMI incomplete media and complete media (10 ml, 2 times). Finally, the pellet was resuspended in 2 ml RPMI complete media and cells were counted using a hemocytometer. Briefly, an aliquot of 10 μl from the suspended cells was added to 90 μl of sterile PBS and 10 μl of this suspension was mixed thoroughly with 10 μl of trypan blue. The mixed suspension was loaded carefully onto the

Neubauer's chamber and all the cells were counted (a non- viable cell stains blue, a viable cell will be opaque). The average of the four quadrates was used for cell counting.

Number of cells/ml = Mean no. of the cells × Dilution factor × 10^4

In-vitro Stimulation of Splenocytes

The splenocytes from each mouse (1×10^6 cells/ well) were suspended in a 24-well tissue culture plate in triplicates. The cultures were stimulated with different doses of CHIK-VLPs (10 µg, 20 µg and 40 µg) corresponding to their designated groups. Concanavalin A (Con A, 5µg/ml; Sigma, USA) as positive control and negative control (without antigen) were also included for each group. The plates were incubated at 37^0C in a 5% CO2 humidified incubator. The culture supernatants were collected from the wells every 24 hrs of *in vitro* stimulation and frozen prior to analysis of specific cytokine. The culture supernatant of frozen splenocytes was centrifuged at 15,000g for 30 minutes at 4^0C; the supernatant was diluted in sterile PBS and assayed for cytokines by the mouse-specific sandwich ELISA kit.

Sandwich ELISA

The expression level of cytokines *i.e.,* TNF-α, IFN-γ, IL-2, IL-4, IL-6 and IL-10 from the culture supernatants of splenocytes of CHIK-VLPs immunized mice and mock immunized mice were measured by Sandwich ELISA using BD OptEIA Kit, (BD Biosciences, USA) according to the manufacturer's instructions.

Preparation of cytokine standards

An aliquot of the standard recombinant cytokine, stored at -80^0C was thawed carefully at RT. Serially two fold dilutions were prepared in the assay diluents for different cytokines *viz.* IL-2 (200 pg/ml-3.1 pg/ml), IL-4 (500 pg/ml-7.8 pg/ml), IL-10 (2000 pg/ml-31.3 pg/ml), IFN-γ (200 pg/ml-31.3 pg/ml), TNF-α (1000 pg/ml-15.6 pg/ml).

Mouse cytokine Sandwich ELISA

Briefly, microtiter plates were coated with capture antibody (100 µl/well) diluted in coating buffer in the triplicates wells, sealed and incubated overnight at 4⁰C. The plates were washed thrice with PBS and blocked with assay diluents (300 μl/well) for 1 hr at RT. The wells were washed 3 times with PBS and PBS-T each and then incubated with standards and culture supernatant samples (100 μl/well) for 2 hrs at RT. The plates were washed 5 times with PBS-T, inverted and blotted on absorbent paper to remove any residual buffer. The plates were then incubated with biotinylated anti-mouse detector monoclonal antibody for 1 hr at RT. The plates were washed 5 times with PBS-T and incubated for 30 min at RT with streptavidin–horseradish peroxidase conjugate (SAv- HRP). The plates were again washed 7 times with PBS-T and PBS and developed with tetramethylbenzidine (TMB) and H_2O_2 for 30 min at RT in dark. The reaction was stopped with 1N H_2SO_4 and the absorbance was read at 450nm. The expression levels of cytokines were determined with the help of a standard curve and presented as picograms per milliliter (pg/ml).

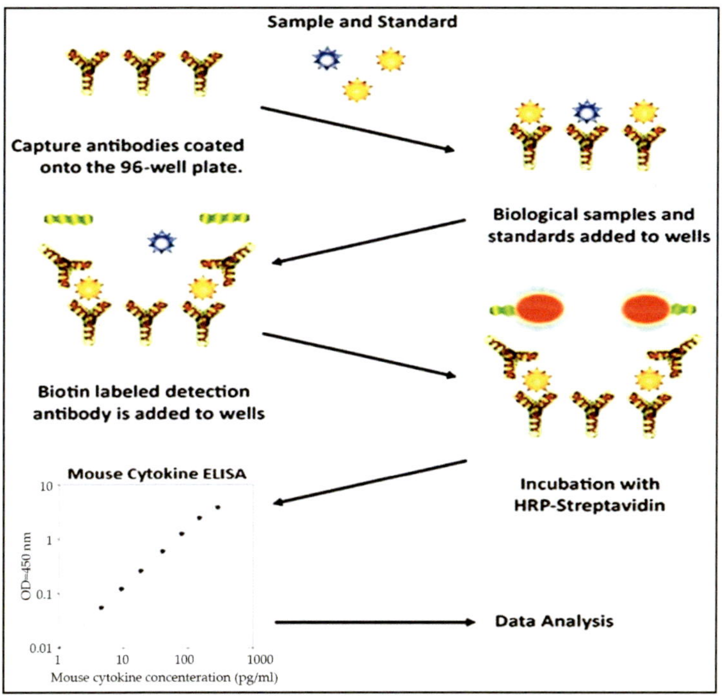

Figure 4.5: Schematic representation of Mouse cytokine Sandwich ELISA.

Statistical Analysis

Statistical comparisons for sample evaluation, antibody titer, IgG isotypes and cytokine levels were done using GraphPad Prism 6 software (La Jolla,

CA), by one-way ANOVA using Multiple Comparison Procedure (Fisher LSD Method). Statistical analyses of serum viremia and body weight gain were performed using an unpaired t-test. Survival curve analysis (percentage survivals) was done by Kaplan Meier's method. Differences were considered to be statistically significant at $P < 0.05$.

CHAPTER 5

EXPRESSION AND CHARACTERIZATION OF CHIKUNGUNYA VIRUS-LIKE PARTICLES AND CONFIRMATION THROUGH MOLECULAR BASED TECHNOLOGY

A TWO-STEP PURIFICATION STRATEGY FOR CHIKUNGUNYA VIRION USING SUCROSE BUOYANT DENSITY GRADIENT SEPARATION

Chikungunya virus has emerged as one of the most important and widespread arboviral infections of public significance. Its recent emergence in both old and new worlds generated immense interest among global researchers to develop suitable diagnostic and medical control measures.

Virus purification is one of the most challenging areas for the development of any downstream research including the development of diagnostics and vaccines. An improved method for purifying the Chikungunya virus from the cell culture supernatant of infected African Green Monkey Kidney (Vero) cells is described. It employs a combination of polyethylene glycol (PEG-6000) precipitation with sucrose gradient ultracentrifugation. The infected cell culture supernatant was precipitated using polyethylene glycol and concentrated virus was banded at the interface of 20-60% (w/v) discontinuous sucrose gradient using rate zonal ultracentrifugation. Using a combination of SDS-PAGE and western blotting techniques, Chikungunya virus structural proteins were detected only in the fractions collected from the interface. The authenticity of the purified Chikungunya virions was further confirmed by reverse transcription polymerase chain reaction (RT-PCR) and transmission electron microscopic (TEM) study.

The developed method has immense application and is useful in making a large quantity of purified Chikungunya virus for its characterization, virus morphological study and purification of Chikungunya Virus-Like particles expressed from the heterologous system.

Chikungunya Virus Propagation and Characterization

The Chikungunya virus (DRDE-07) used in the present study was propagated in Vero cells. Viral growth kinetics was studied at 24 hr intervals in Vero cells by plaque assay and by real time RT-PCR and it was found that virus titer was highest at 2 days post-infection (dpi) (Fig.5.1 a & b). Microscopic analysis showed a prominent cytopathic effect (CPE) at 48 hpi (Fig 5.1 a). This was also confirmed by immunofluorescence (Fig 5.2 b). Further the virus titer was increased by repeated passaging and finally obtained titer was 2.3 X 10^8 pfu/ml (Fig 5.3). This high titered virus was produced in bulk volume for further experiments.

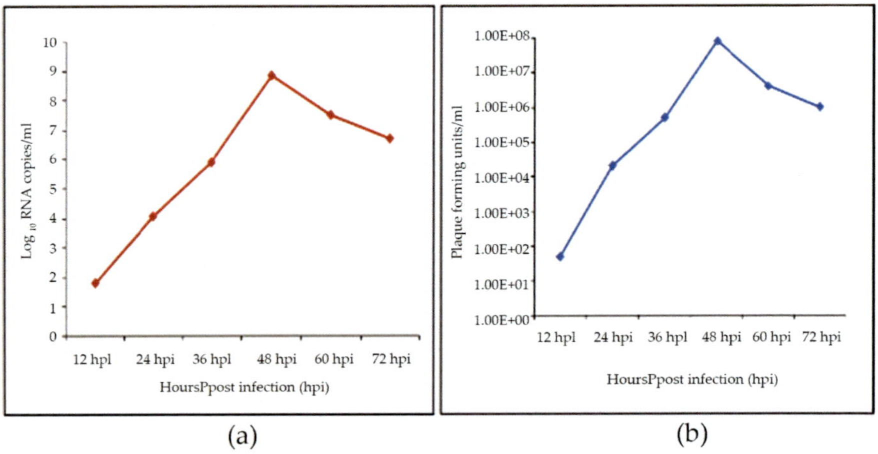

Figure 5.1: Titer of Chikungunya infected Vero cells at 24 hr intervals i.e. from 1 dpi to 3 dpi in terms of (a) Log_{10} RNA copies/ml (b) Plaque forming unit (PFU) titer/ml.

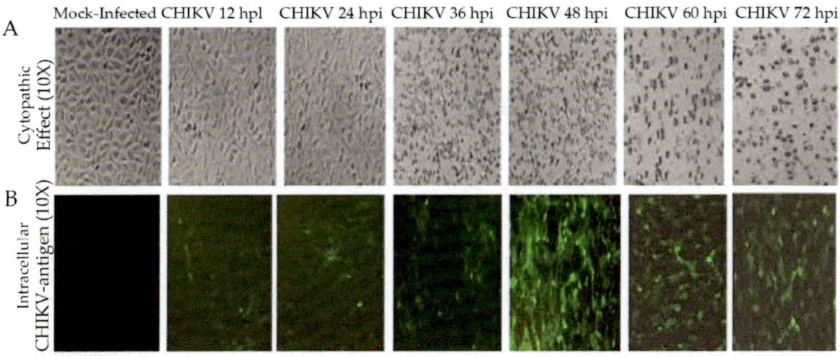

Figure 5.2: Morphological changes in CHIKV infected Vero cells. Cells were infected with CHIKV and analyzed for cytopathic effect (panel A) and presence of intracellular CHIKV antigen (panel B). Panel A shows the morphological representation of CHIKV-induced CPE at 10X magnification showing the appearance of rounded and dense cells. Panel B represents the percentage of total fluorescence positive cells at 10X size. For all the above parameters, microscopic counting was done in 5 different microscopic zones and values are given as mean.

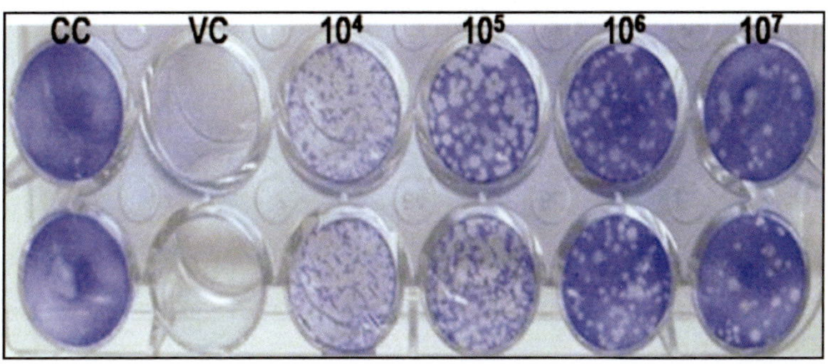

Figure 5.3: Titration of Chikungunya virus by plaque assay where the virus is serially 10-fold diluted and the test is performed in duplicate (CC- cell control, VC- virus control).

Purification of Chikungunya Virus by Density Gradient Centrifugation

Vero cells grown in 225 cm^2 flasks up to 80-90% confluency were infected with Chikungunya virus. The virus titer was highest at 2 dpi as shown in the virus growth kinetics study. So at 2 dpi, the cell supernatant was harvested and centrifuged at 1000xg for 15 min at 4^{0}C. Plaque assay confirmed the presence of a high titered virus of 10^8 PFU/ml. Then, polyethylene glycol (PEG-6000) was used for concentrating the virus particles by precipitation, further sucrose density gradient ultracentrifugation resulted in the formation of a native virus antigen layer in between the two sucrose concentrations (Fig 5.4a).

SDS-PAGE analysis of different fractions revealed that the majority of chikungunya virions are localized in the 20-60% sucrose interface (Fig. 5.4a). The envelope glycoproteins E1 and E2 of CHIKV migrate very close to one another on the SDS-PAGE gel and form a single band at the region corresponding to ~55 kDa (Fig. 5.4b). The capsid protein was seen as a separate band at the region corresponding to the size of ~32 kDa. However, the band corresponding to the size of E3 was not visible on the SDS-PAGE gel.

In order to examine the authenticity of the purified virus, different fractions collected from the buoyant density gradient were analyzed *via* western blotting using Chikungunya envelope protein (E2) specific polyclonal antibodies. As seen in (Fig-5.4c), the E2 protein was recognized by the specific antibodies only from the 20-60% interface band and the fractions that were very close to the interface.

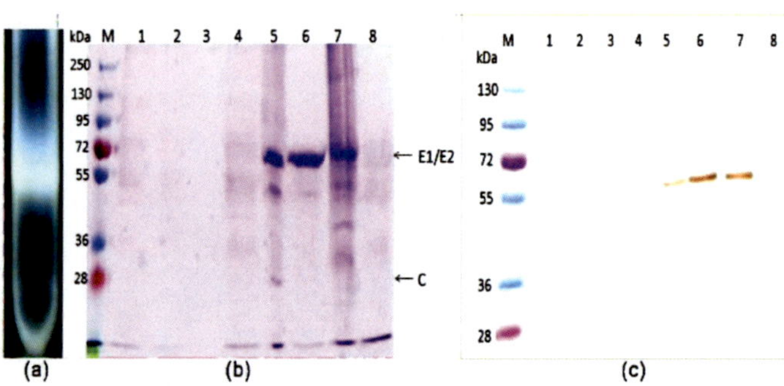

Figure 5.4: Purification of Chikungunya virus: (a) Separated fractions of Chikungunya virus-infected culture supernatant in Sucrose density gradient centrifugation; (b) SDS- PAGE analysis of purified Chikungunya virus fractions from discontinuous sucrose gradient; (c) Western blot analysis of purified Chikungunya virus fractions. Lane M: prestained molecular weight marker (Fermentas, USA); Lanes 1-4: fractions collected from 20% sucrose layer; Lane 5: fraction slightly above 20-60% interface; Lane 6: band collected from 20-60% interface; Lane 7: fraction collected slightly below 20-60% interface, Lane 8: fraction from 60% sucrose layer.

CONFIRMATION OF PURIFIED CHIKUNGUNYA VIRUS THROUGH REVERSE TRANSCRIPTION-POLYMERASE CHAIN REACTION (RT-PCR)

The genomic RNA obtained from the 20-60% interface band amplified the partial region of CHIKV polyprotein through RT-PCR (Fig 4.5) which results in a band of 1795 bp corresponding partial 5' region of the polyprotein encoding gene thus confirming the authenticity of the purified virions.

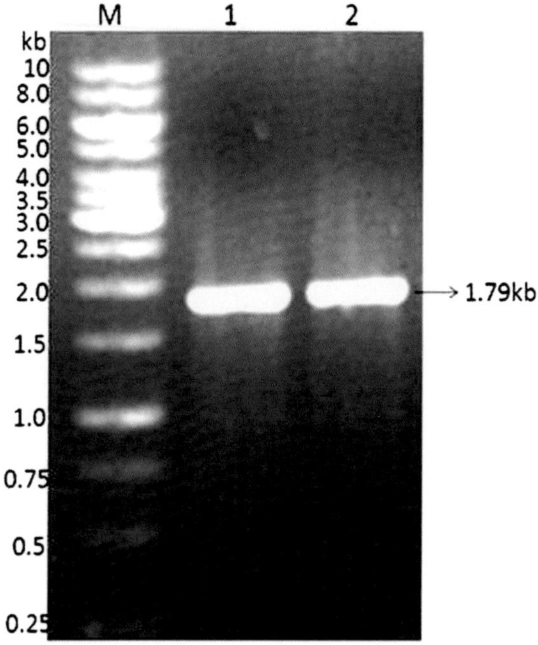

Figure 5.5: Confirmation of purified Chikungunya Virus through reverse Transcription-polymerase chain reaction (RT-PCR); Lane M: GeneRuler 1 kb DNA Ladder (Fermentas, USA); Lane 1-2: Amplification from purified Chikungunya virus collected from the 20-60% interface.

Transmission Electron Microscopy (TEM) Analysis

The negative staining of the fraction collected from the 20-60% interface band revealed the presence of both cores and complete virions under the transmission electron microscope (Fig. 5.6). The average diameter of Chikungunya cores was approximately 40 nm and complete virions had varied sized particles ranging from 50-65 nm.

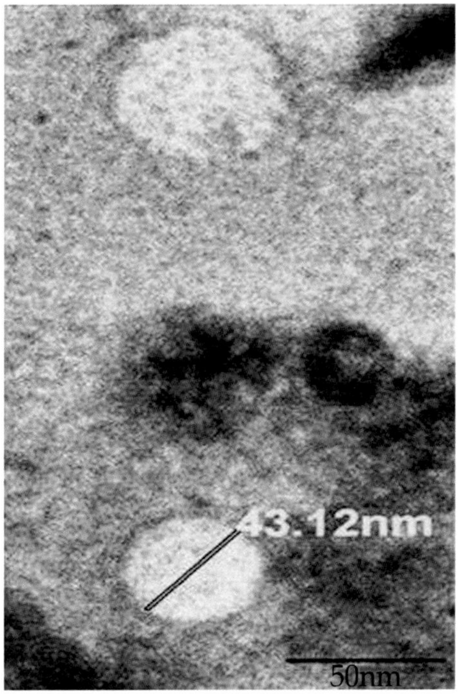

Figure 5.6: Negatively stained Chikungunya virions as seen under the transmission electron microscope (Scale bar, 50 nm).

Virus purification is a crucial method for several downstream applications and hence it is necessary to have an easy and simplified method that gives consistent results. In the present study, we report a two-step method for purifying the Chikungunya virus from the infected cell culture supernatant. The procedure involves a combination of virus precipitation using polyethylene glycol-6000 and virus concentration using sucrose density gradient ultracentrifugation. Chikungunya viral particles could be banded at the interface of 20-60% (w/v) discontinuous sucrose gradient using rate zonal ultra centrifugation. Upon electrophoresis of the purified virus, on denaturing PAGE, E1/ E2 bands corresponding to the size of ~55 kDa and Capsid protein of size ~32 kDa were noticed. As reported earlier, the association between E1 and E2 of CHIKV is very strong than any other related alphaviruses and it was very difficult to separate E1 from E2 on electrophoresis (Simizu et al., 1984). The observed finding is in accordance with the earlier reports (Pedersen et al., 1974; Konishi et al., 1980). There was a slight increase in the size of E1/E2 proteins due to the presence of sucrose in the virus preparation which makes the protein have slightly retarded movement.

The obtained size of the capsid protein is in agreement with that of the earlier reports (Akahata et al., 2010; Sourisseau et al., 2007). In the present study, no other proteins were noticed smaller than the capsid protein and the band intensity of capsid protein was weak in comparison to the E1/E2 protein as also reported by Simizu, et al. (1984). Our study also suggests that the E3 of CHIKV is not associated with the virions and is released into infected culture fluids, which is in agreement with the previous report (Simizu, et al., 1984) and hence is not visible on the SDS-PAGE gel.

The authenticity of the virus protein in the purified fraction was reconfirmed *via* western blotting using envelope protein (E2) specific antibodies. From our results, it is evident that the 20-60% sucrose gradient is efficient as the Chikungunya virus could not penetrate the 60% sucrose layer. The top 20% sucrose layer was sufficient enough to selectively permit the Chikungunya virions while arresting other media or host cell-derived proteins.

The present study is of significant importance, as we have successfully used PEG-6000 to concentrate and reduce the volume of low titer virus for ultracentrifugation. In addition, earlier studies by Eckels et al., 1970, have used multiple steps that involve initial high-speed ultracentrifugation and tween ether extraction for virus concentration followed by sucrose gradients (5-30% in PBS) for purifying the CHIKV virus. As the use of multiple steps and detergents may damage the virions, we have developed an improved method with only two steps for better purification of CHIKV with minimum impurities. Both cores with an approximate diameter of 40 nm and complete virions of diameter 50-65 nm were seen on the transmission electron microscope. This observation is in agreement with that of a recent study by Akahata, et al 2010, where Chiknungunya Virus-Like particles (CHIK-VLPs) have been analyzed by Cryo electron microscopy and three-dimensional image reconstruction wherein the VLPs had an external diameter of 65 nm and a core diameter of 40 nm. This purification strategy can be utilized for efficient purification of CHIKV virion or Virus-Like particles (VLPs) required for other downstream applications.

HETEROLOGOUS EXPRESSION AND CHARACTERIZATION OF CHIK-VLPS USING PICHIA PASTORIS

Chikungunya virus (CHIKV) is becoming a global concern due to the increasing number of outbreaks throughout the world and the absence of any CHIKV-specific vaccine or treatment. There is also a scarcity of reliable diagnostic kits in endemic areas, making disease management extremely difficult. Virus-like particles (VLPs) are multistructured proteins that mimic the organization and conformation of native viruses but lack the viral genome.

Therefore, they are noninfectious and potentially safer vaccine candidates and diagnostic antigens. Previously, CHIK-VLPs have been expressed in mammalian and baculovirus insect cell expression systems and found to be effective as vaccine candidates. But these VLPs have some disadvantages; CHIK-VLPs based on mammalian cell expression systems are primarily related to higher production costs. Moreover, in the baculovirus insect cell expression system, co-production of enveloped baculovirus particles contaminates the vaccine candidate and may impair the vaccine quality. Moreover, baculovirus particles and VLPs are difficult to separate; VLPs produced in this system have to undergo either chemical inactivation treatments or several downstream processing steps to eliminate baculovirus infectivity that subsequently increasing the production cost.

The *Pichia pastoris* (*P. pastoris*) yeast expression system used in this study offers several advantages for VLPs development: the techniques needed for molecular manipulation are simple, the ability to produce large-scale foreign proteins in their native conformation, using simple chemical media make it an attractive alternative platform. Further, the *Pichia* cell can grow to high density in suspension culture improving the productivity of this platform. Recent studies demonstrated that CHIK-VLPs have antigenic specificity which was similar to native CHIKV. We transformed the GS115 strain of *Pichia pastoris* with the yeast transfer vector having the C-E3-E2-6k-E1 gene and optimized its expression parameters *viz.* different concentration of methanol, culture medium and time of VLP harvest. We detected 50 kDa protein corresponding to E1 and/or E2 in the supernatant. Transmission electron microscopy revealed spherical particles with a 50- to 60-nm diameter in the supernatant that resembled the native CHIKV virions. The yield of purified VLPs was 60 ng/μl. These VLPs were shown to react with serum raised against CHIKV-E2 protein, indicating that their antigenicity is similar to that of native CHIKV. These results indicated that CHIK-VLPs are morphologically and antigenically similar to the native CHIKV, suggesting that they have the potential for use in chikungunya diagnostic and vaccine formulation.

CLONING OF THE CHIKV POLYPROTEIN GENE OF CHIKUNGUNYA VIRUS IN PTZ57 T/A CLONING VECTOR

Gene coding for ORF of structural Polyprotein of Chikungunya virus was cloned as left and right fragments in the pTZ57R/T T/A cloning vector.

Amplification of CHIKV Polyprotein Gene by One Step RT-PCR

The gene encoding CHIKV polyprotein was amplified as two fragments known as left and right fragments having *XhoI* natural restriction site. The conventional RT-PCR was performed with the above-mentioned primer sets targeting the left and right fragments of the CHIKV polyprotein gene. The size of the amplified product was analyzed by 1% agarose gel electrophoresis and was compared with a standard DNA marker. Distinct single DNA bands of 1.795 Kbp and 1.952 Kbp size were observed corresponding Right and Left fragments of CHIKV structural polyprotein gene (Fig. 5.7) with reaction conditions mentioned under material and methods, Hence these conditions were considered to be optimal and were used for subsequent amplifications. The PCR product was purified and the concentration of purified DNA was estimated to be approximately 150ng/μl.

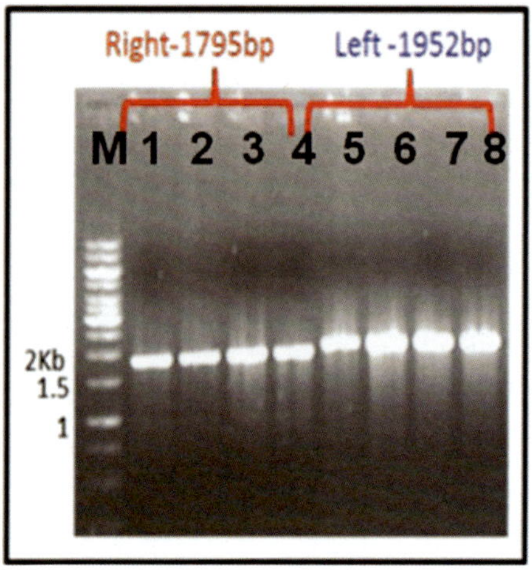

Figure 5.7: RT-PCR of PCR CHIKV structural polyprotein gene as Right and Left fragment; Lane M: GeneRuler 1 Kb DNA Ladder (Fermentas, USA); Lane 1-4: Amplified Right fragment of CHIKV structural polyprotein gene; Lane 5-8: Amplified Left fragment of CHIKV structural polyprotein gene.

CONSTRUCTION OF PTZ57-LEFT AND PTZ57-RIGHT CONSTRUCT IN DH5-A CELLS

For constructing pTZ57-Left and pTZ57-Right construct, these amplified products were ligated with the pTZ57 T/A cloning vector. The ligated construct was then transformed into DH5-α cells *via* heat shock method. Clones were screened by colony lysis method (Fig. 5.8a & 5.7b). In colony lysis screening, constructs that were showing slower mobility indicate their higher molecular weight and may be assumed as positive construct. Then these clones were grown and their plasmids have been isolated and their authenticity was confirmed by PCR analysis (Fig. 5.9).

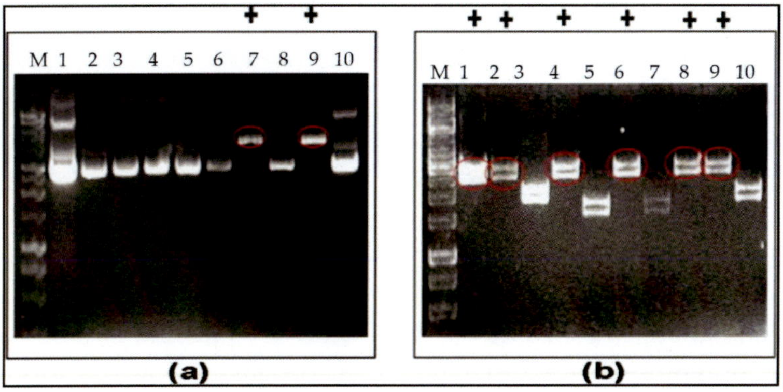

Figure 5.8: Colony lysis Screening of the CHIKV structural polyprotein**;** Left (a) and Right (b) clones into pTZ57 T/A cloning vector Lane M: GeneRuler 1 Kb DNA Ladder (Fermentas, USA); Lane 1-10: Crude plasmid of different clones; +: Running higher may be positive clones.

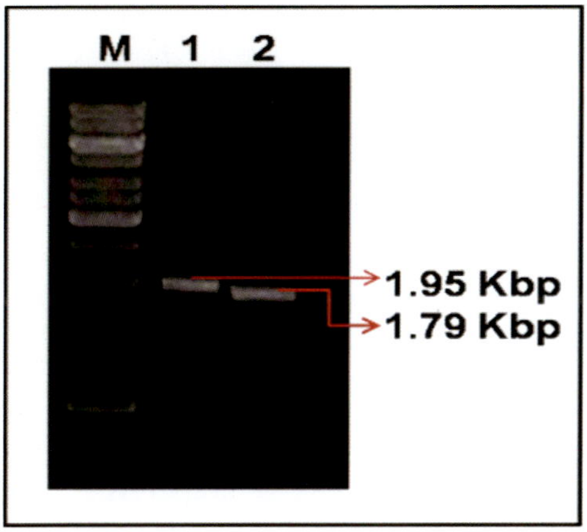

Figure 5.9: PCR amplification of pTZ57Left and of pTZ57 Right clones; M-1Kb DNA ladder; Lane 1- Positive clone having the left fragment of CHIKV structural polyprotein gene; Lane 2- Positive clone having the right fragment of CHIKV structural polyprotein gene.

Construction of pTZ57-C-E3-E2-6K-E1 Construct in DH5-α Cells

CHIKV structural polyprotein gene was cloned as left and right fragments in the pTZ57 vector. For constructing the full length of the CHIKV polyprotein gene both the construct having left and right fragments was digested by using *XbaI* & *XhoI* restriction enzymes, which resulted in 1.9 Kbp release from pTZ57Left and 4 Kbp linearized pTZ57 Right construct (Fig. 5.10a & b). Now both the insert and vector were ligated and transformed into DH5-α cells to construct pTZ57-C-E3-E2-6K-E1 plasmid having complete structural polyprotein gene of CHIKV. The construct hence formed was confirmed by colony lysis (Fig. 5.11a). Further, the clones were also confirmed by restriction digestion analysis using *XbaI* enzyme where the respective inserts were released from the recombinant vector (Fig. 5.11b).

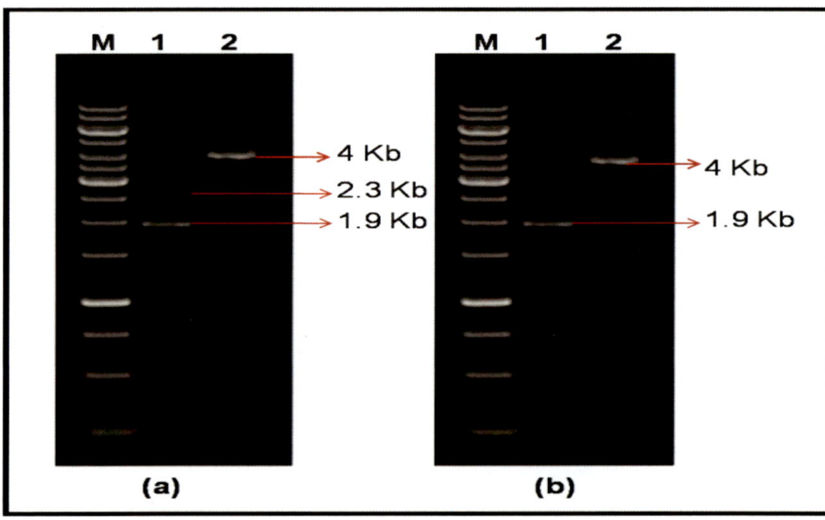

Figure 5.10: Digestion of pTZ57 Left and of pTZ57 Right clones with *XhoI and XbaI*, (a). Released left fragment and linearized pTZ57 Right plasmid; M- 1Kb DNA ladder; Lane 1- Digested Positive clone having the left fragment of CHIKV structural polyprotein gene; Lane 2- Digested Positive clone having the right fragment of CHIKV structural polyprotein gene. (b) Purified left (insert) and pTZ57 Right vector. M- 1Kb DNA ladder; Lane 1- Purified left insert Lane 2- Purified right vector.

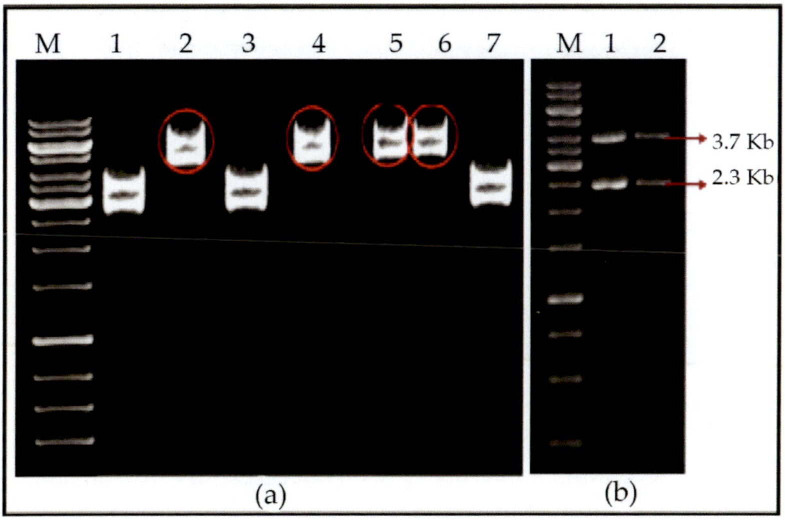

Figure 5.11: Screening of pTZ57-C-E3-E2-6K-E1 recombinant plasmids. (a). Colony lysis Screening of CHIKV structural polyprotein clones into pTZ57 T/A cloning vector; M- 1Kb DNA ladder; Lane 1-7 crude plasmid from different colonies; Lane 2,4,5,6- Recombinant clone may be positive. (b) Restriction digestion of positive recombinant clones. M-1Kb DNA ladder; Lane 1-2 digested plasmid from positive recombinant clones 1 and 2.

Sub Cloning of CHIKV Polyprotein Gene into the pPIC9K Yeast Transfer Vector

The full CHIKV polyprotein gene was cloned in the pTZ57 vector. For constructing the pPIC9K-ChikV-C-E3-E2-6K-E1 transfer vector, the full structural polyprotein Chikungunya virus was amplified from the pTZ57-C-E3-E2-6K-E1 construct by using CHIKYVLP forward and CHIKYVLP reverse primers. Chikungunya virus having the 3.7 Kbp long DNA fragment encoding CHIKV structural polyprotein gene was amplified using gradient PCR at different annealing temperatures by CHIKYVLP forward and CHIKYVLP reverse primers (Fig. 5.12a). 58^{0}C temperature was found to be optimum for amplifying the structural polyprotein gene. Further CHIKV structural polyprotein gene was amplified at 58^{0}C annealing temperature (Fig. 4.12b) and cloned into the pPIC9K yeast expression vector (Fig 5.13a) The positive clones were confirmed by colony lysis (Fig 5.13b), PCR analysis (Fig. 4.13c) and restriction analysis by using *AvrII* and *SnaBI* restriction enzymes (Fig 5.13d).

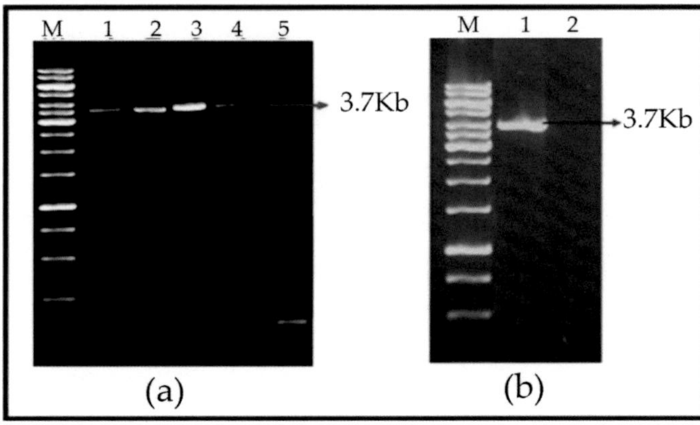

Figure 5.12: PCR amplification of CHIKV structural polyprotein gene; (a) Optimization of PCR amplification of CHIKV structural polyprotein gene at different temperature;M- DNA ladder (Fermentas #SM1163);1,2, 3, 4- PCR amplicon from pTZ57- C/E3/E2/6K/E1 construct at different temperature (54, 56, 58 and 62^{0}C); 5- Negative control (NTC) (b) PCR amplification of CHIKV C-E3-E2-6K-E1 proteins gene at optimized temperature; M- DNA ladder (Fermentas #SM1163); Lane1-PCR amplicon from pTZ57C/E3/E2/6K/E1 construct; Lane 2- Negative control (NTC).

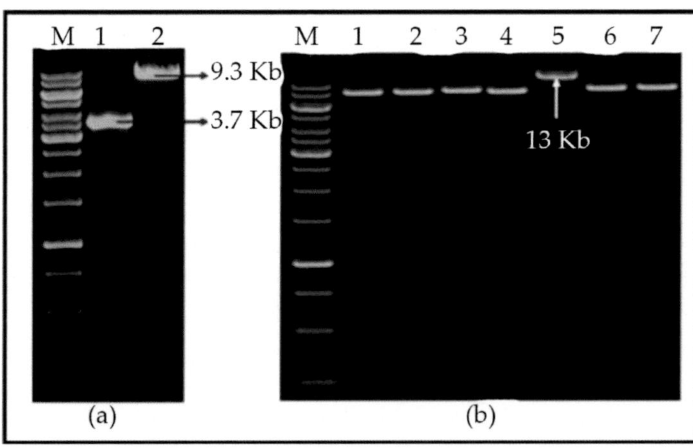

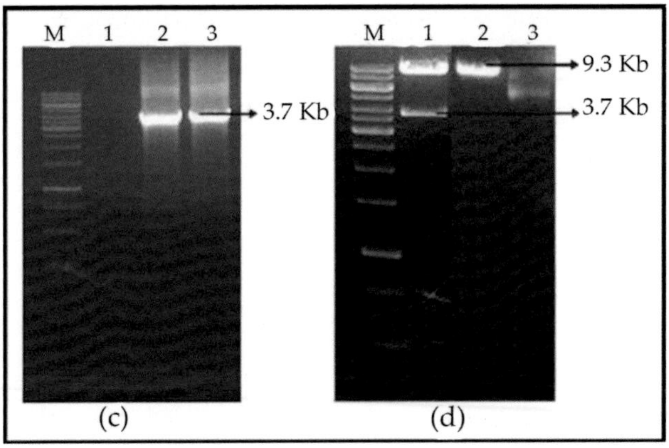

Figure 5.13: Cloning of Structural polyprotein in pPIC9K yeast transfer vector; (a) Linearization of PCR product and vector with *SnaB*I and *Avr*II; M- DNA ladder, 1- Linearized PCR amplicon from pTZ57-C/E3/E2/6K/E1 construct, 2- Linerized pPIC9K vector; (b) Rapid screening of transformants through the improved colony lysis method ; M- DNA ladder, 1-7 bacterial cell lysates from colonies, 1 / 7 clones (Lane 5) positive for CHIKV polyprotein insert; (c) PCR analysis of pPIC9KCHIKV C-E3-E2-6K-E1 clone; M- DNA ladder, 1- PCR amplification from pPIC9K plasmid (negative control), 2- PCR amplification from pPICK9K C-E3-E2-6K-E1 clone, 3- PCR amplification from pTZ57- C/E3/E2/6K/E1(positive control); (d) Restriction analysis of recombinant clone; M- DNA ladder, 1- pPIC9KCHIKV C-E3-E2-6K-E1 clone *SnaB* I & *Avr* II *digest,* 2- pPIC9K plasmid control *SnaB* I & *Avr* II *digest*, *3*- pPIC9K plasmid uncut.

Transformation of the pPIC9K-CHIKV-C-E3-E2-6K-E1 recombinant construct into yeast (Pichia pastoris) GS115 strain

LINEARIZATION OF THE PPIC9K-CHIKV-C-E3-E2-6K-E1 CONSTRUCT

Recombinant plasmid pPIC9K-CHIKV-C-E3-E2-6K-E1 carrying full structural polyprotein gene (Fig 5.14a) was isolated. DNA sample thus prepared was quantified using Nanodrop. Upon quantification, the concentration of pPIC9K-CHIKV-C- E3-E2-6K-E1 plasmid DNA was 256ng/µl. The A_{260}/A_{280} ratio was 1.87 for the above plasmid indicating the purity of DNA preparation, which was good enough for the transformation purpose. The recombinant plasmid DNA (~10µg) was linearized by digesting with *Sac* I enzyme to integrate the transgene at the His4 locus on the *Pichia* genome and also to generate HIS $^{+}$ Mut^{+} transformants in *Pichia pastoris* GS115 cells. After digestion, the DNA was purified through QIAquick Gel extraction and visualized on the agarose gel. After *Sac*I digestion single 13 Kbp band was observed on agarose gel (Fig 5.14b).

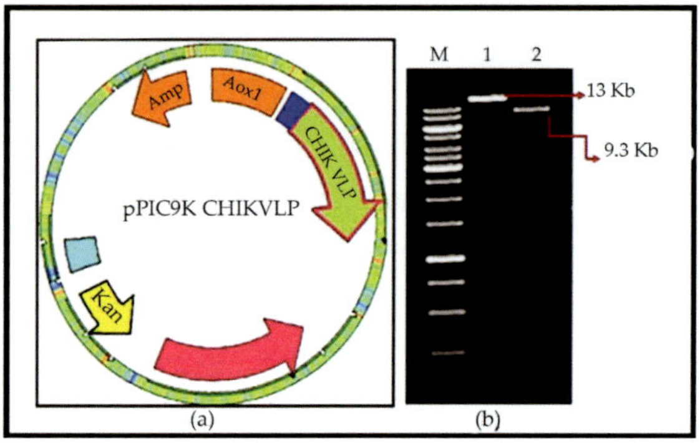

Figure 5.14: Linearization of the pPIC9KCHIKVLP construct; (a) Vector map of the pPIC9KCHIKVLP construct; (b) Linearization of recombinant and non-recombinant plasmid with *Sac*I; M- DNA ladder, 1 - pPICK9K C-E3-E2-6K-E1 Digested with *Sac* I, 2- pPICK9K plasmid Digested with *Sac*I

Optimization of Transformation Voltage

A total of three hundred and sixty-five transformed colonies bearing the chromosomally integrated copies of pPIC9K-CHIKV-C-E3-E2-6K-E1 were obtained on different transformation plates. 80, 231 and 43 colonies were observed with 1600V, 1800V and 2000V respectively. This indicates that 1800V is a good enough voltage to get more transformants.

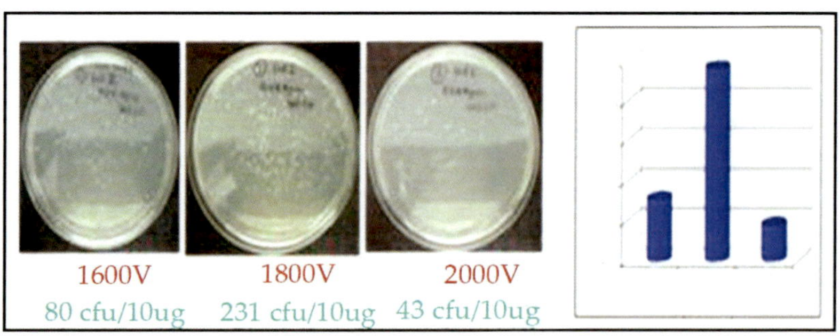

Figure 5.15: Colonies obtained on RD agar plates after transformation at different voltages.

Screening of Positive Transformants (*Pichia* Clone)

Pichia transformants were screened through Geneticin (G418) sensitivity assay and PCR analysis to select the colonies with inserted target DNA.

Geneticin Sensitivity Assay

Colonies obtained on different transformation plates were further screened for single, double or multiple copy integrants through replica plating on YPD plates containing different concentrations of Geneticin (500 μg/ml, 750 μg/ml and 1000 μg/ml). A further selection of all transformants on Geneticin containing YPD plates resulted in 106 colonies showing resistance to different concentrations of Geneticin tested. Forty nine colonies appeared on the plate containing 500μg/ml Geneticin, whereas the selection plates with 750 μg/ml and 1000 μg/ ml Geneticin had 32 and 25 colonies respectively. This indicated that these 25 clones might have multiple copies of the structural polyprotein gene of CHIKV since they were growing on higher antibiotic concentrations.

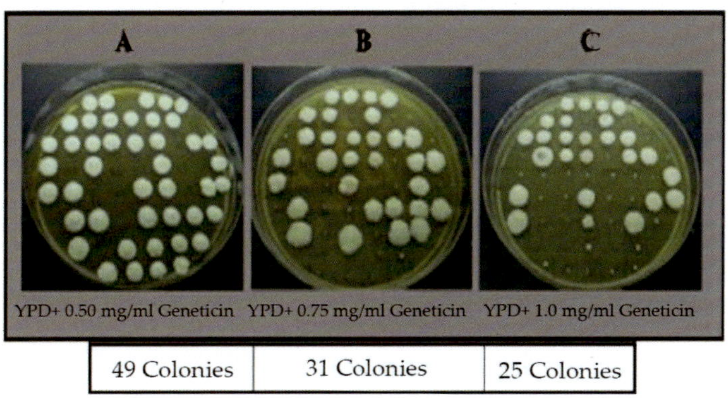

Figure 5.16: Geneticin sensitivity assay for recombinant *Pichia pastoris* having the structural polyprotein gene of Chikungunya virus integrated into genomic DNA.

Genomic DNA PCR Analysis

For preliminary screening of recombinant clones having differential copy numbers of the transgene, a simple PCR was performed using equal concentrations of genomic DNA. For this genomic DNA from recombinant clones was isolated and visualized on 1% agarose gel (Fig. 5.17a). Further genomic DNA was quantified by Nanodrop and 1μg DNA from all samples was used as a template for PCR amplification. Genomic DNA PCR from ten selected yeast transformants using AOX 1 forward and CHIKYVLP reverse primer resulted in amplification of approximately 3.9 Kbp products as expected. Nine out of ten DNA samples amplified the expected 3.9 Kbp DNA along with the known positive control (Fig. 5.17b), whereas, DNA from nonrecombinants did not show any amplification. Multiple copy integrants having more than four copies of structural polyprotein gene were selected based on antibiotic sensitivity assay and genomic DNA PCR. The clones that were resistant to higher concentrations of Geneticin also showed intensive bands in genomic DNA PCR and these results were in agreement with that of the Geneticin sensitivity assay.

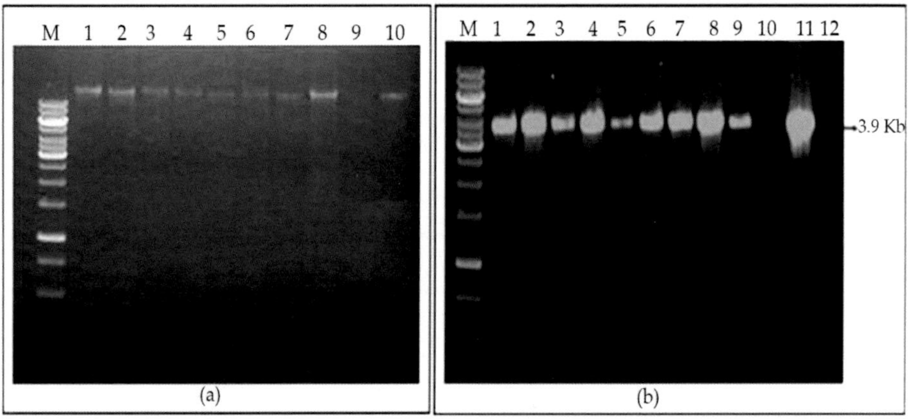

Figure 5.17: Genomic DNA PCR analysis; (a) Agarose gel showing genomic DNA; Lane M- DNA ladder (1 Kb), Lane 1-10 Genomic DNA from selected CHIK-VLPs-*Pichia* transformants; (b) Genomic DNA PCR confirmation of transgene integration in CHIKVLPs-*Pichia* transformants; Lane M- DNA ladder (1 Kb), Lane 1-10 PCR amplification from genomic DNA, Lane 11- PCR amplification from p pPIC9K-CHIKV- C-E3-E2-6K-E1 plasmid DNA (Positive control), Lane 12- NTC.

Expression of Recombinant CHIK-VLPs

Eight colonies that were found positive with PCR having different copy numbers of the transgene were selected for induction and their expression level was checked in denaturing conditions. Out of eight PCR-positive clones, seven clones were found to express a 50 kDa protein band (around) that corresponds to the size of E1 and E2 proteins of Chikungunya virus (fig 5.18). This expression was also confirmed by anti-E2 antibodies.

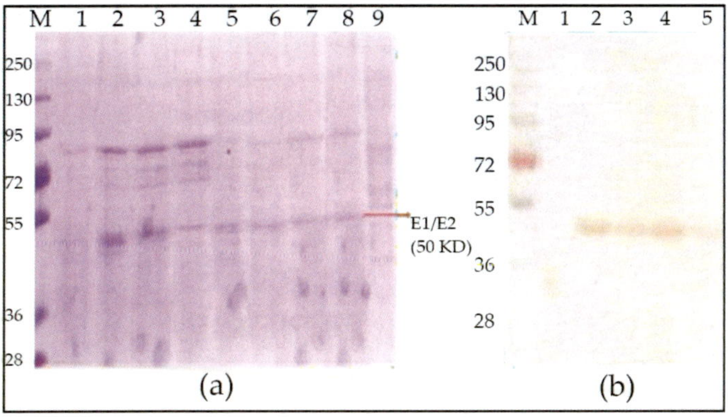

Figure 5.18: Expression profile of different recombinant *Pichia* clones at denaturing condition. (a) SDS-PAGE analysis of different clones expressing CHIK-VLPs; Lane M- protein marker (Fermentas SM1811); Lane 1-8 expression profile of different clones at 48 hrs; Lane 9 -Negative control (*Pichia* transformed with pPICK9K without insert) (b) Western blot of different clones expressing CHIK-VLPs; Lane 1- Negative control; Lane 2-5 supernatant of different CHIK-VLPs expressing clones.

Methanol Optimization

PCR positive His^+ Mut^+ *Pichia* clone that was showing resistance at higher antibiotic concentrations was selected for methanol induction. Several methanol concentrations ranging from 0.5 to 2.5% (0.5%, 1%, 1.5%, 2% and 2.5%) were tried in order to choose the optimum concentration of methanol for induction in case of shake flask culture. Incubation was continued at 28^0C on an orbitary shaker (200 rpm) for 96 hrs. Expression of recombinant protein was found to increase with increasing methanol concentration. However, no increase in the expression level was observed at a methanol concentration of >2%. Thus, the optimum methanol concentration for better expression of CHIK-VLPs was found to be 2 %. The expressed protein yield was shown to increase up to 48 hrs post induction after this time point, protein concentration was stable that shows, 48 hrs is the optimum time to harvest CHIK-VLPs (Fig. 5.19)

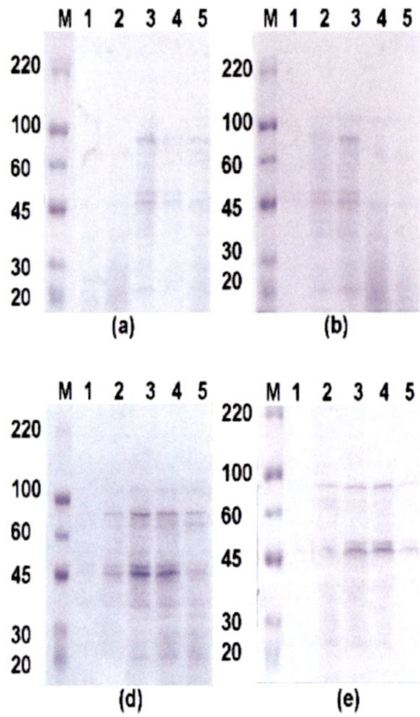

Figure 5.19: Methanol optimization of *Pichia* clone expressing CHIK-VLPs. (a) SDS- PAGE with 0.5% methanol induction; (b) SDS-PAGE with 1% methanol induction; (c) SDS-PAGE with 1.5% methanol induction; (d) SDS-PAGE with 2% methanol induction; (e) SDS-PAGE with 2.5% methanol induction; Lane M- Prestained protein marker (Sigma); Lane 1- uninduced fraction; Lane 2- 24 hrs fraction; Lane 3- 48 hrs fraction; Lane 4- 72 hrs fraction; Lane 5- 96 hrs fraction.

MEDIA OPTIMIZATION OF CHIK-VLPS EXPRESSION IN THE *PICHIA* SYSTEM

For selecting an optimum medium to obtain the maximum yield of expressed CHIK-VLPs two different media YPGy and BMGM were used for initial culture growth and YPM and BMM with 2% methanol were used for induction. Protein expression in the case of each medium after induction with 2% methanol is shown in fig. 5.20. The expression of CHIK-VLPs appeared to be better in the case of YPM (Fig. 5.20b). Cultures were analyzed for optical density at a wavelength of 600 nm (A_{600}) once every 6 h.

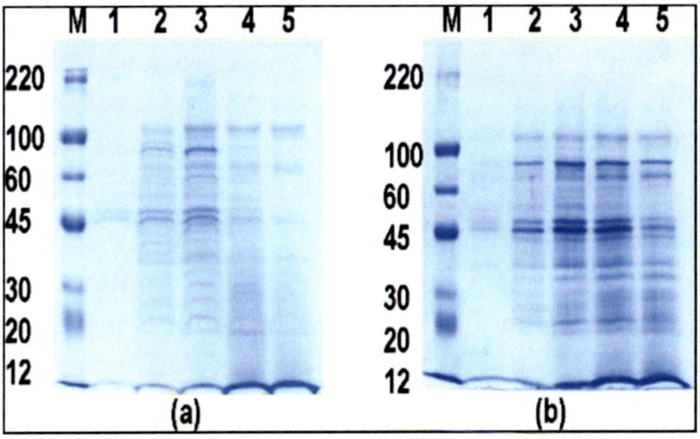

Figure 5.20: Media optimization of Pichia clone expressing CHIK-VLPs. (a) SDS- PAGE profile of recombinant *Pichia pastoris* in BMM; (b) SDS-PAGE profile of recombinant *Pichia pastoris* in YPM; Lane M- Protein marker (Sigma); Lane 1 Negative control, lane 2-5 Fraction from different time points (24 hrs- 96 hrs).

Concentration of Yeast Derived CHIK-VLPs

The structural polyprotein of CHIKV was fused with the α- factor secretion signal of *Saccharomyces cerevisiae* under the control of methanol inducible *Pichia pastoris* alcohol oxidase 1 (AOX1) promoter in the pPIC9K yeast transfer vector. This α-factor secretion signal helps in secreted expression. Hence, CHIK-VLPs were secreted in the culture medium. Purification by ultracentrifugation needs a concentrated sample. The concentration of CHIK-VLPs was done *via* a 10 kDa cutoff membrane filter at 5000 rpm for 30 min.

Purification of the Yeast Derived CHIK-VLPs by Ultracentrifugation

The concentrated protein sample was subjected to ultra-centrifugation. Concentrated CHIK-VLPs were layered over a discontinuous sucrose gradient and centrifuged in a TH-641 swinging bucket rotor (Thermo Scientific, USA) for 16 h at 35,000 rpm at 4^{0}C. Further sucrose density gradient ultracentrifugation resulted in the formation of an opaque layer in between the two sucrose concentrations (Fig 5.21a).

SDS-PAGE analyses of different fractions revealed that the majority of CHIK-VLPs are localized at the 20-60% sucrose interface (Fig. 5.21a). As seen in (Fig-5.21b), envelope glycoproteins E1 and E2 of CHIKV migrate very close to one another on the SDS-PAGE gel and form a single band at the region corresponding to ~55 kDa. The Capsid protein was seen as a separate band at the region corresponding to the size of ~32 kDa. No band corresponding to the size of E3 was visible on the SDS-PAGE gel.

In order to examine the authenticity of the CHIK-VLPs, different fractions collected from the buoyant density gradient were analyzed *via* western blotting using Chikungunya envelope protein (E2) specific antibodies (Fig.5.21c), anti-E1 antibodies and also by using anti-CHIKV antibodies (Fig.5.22).

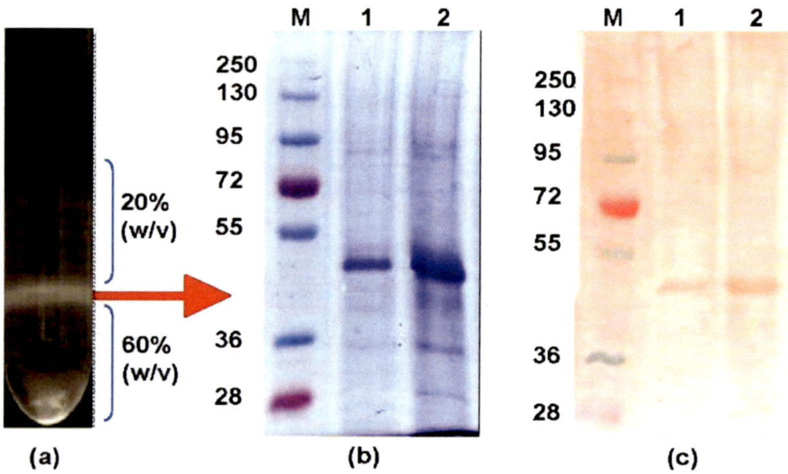

Figure 5.21: Purification and characterization of Chikungunya Virus-Like particles: (a) Separated interface fractions of Chikungunya Virus-Like particles in sucrose density gradient centrifugation; (b) SDS-PAGE analysis of purified Chikungunya Virus-Like particles from discontinuous sucrose gradient; (c) Western blot analysis of purified Chikungunya virus fractions. Lane M: prestained molecular weight marker (Fermentas, USA); Lane 1: Just above Interface; Lane 2: Interface (20-60%).

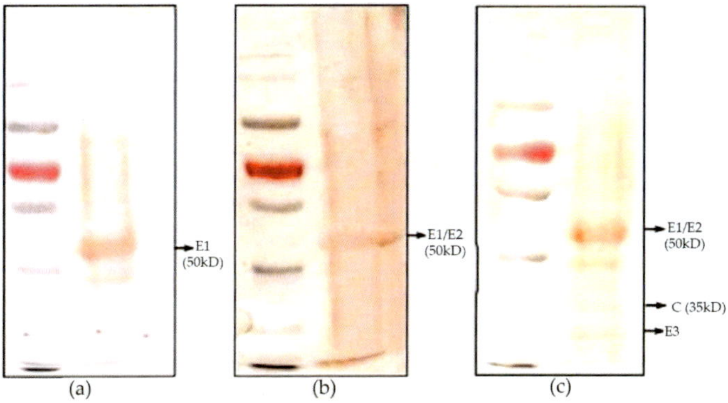

Figure 5.22: Characterization of VLPs *via* Immuno-blotting using different CHIKV-specific antibodies: (a) Western blot using anti-E1 mAb; (b) WB using anti-E2 pAb; (c) WB using anti-native CHIKV pAb.

TRANSMISSION ELECTRON MICROSCOPY (TEM) ANALYSIS OF PURIFIED CHIK-VLPS

The negative staining of the fraction collected from the 20-60% interface band revealed the presence of spherical particles of approximately 65-70 nm under the t transmission electron microscope (Fig. 5.23). The average diameter of Chikungunya cores was approximately 40 nm. Electron microscopy showed that the VLPs had an external diameter of 65 nm and a core diameter of 40 nm which is consistent with the reported size (65-70 nm) of the chikungunya virus and other alphaviruses.

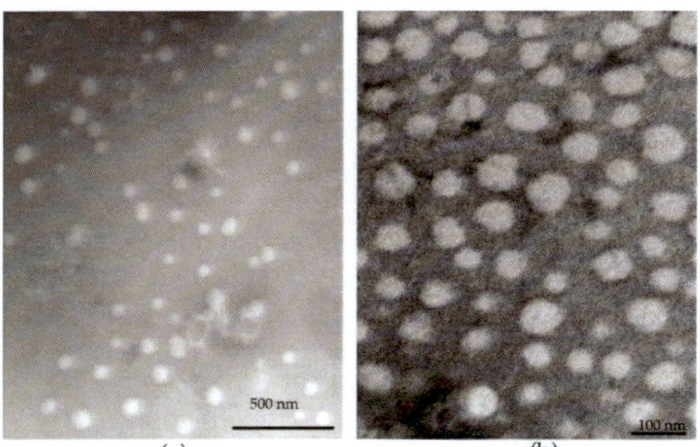

Figure 5.23: Transmission electron microscopy analysis of purified CHIK-VLPs: (a) Electron micrograph of purified CHIK-VLPs at 40,000 X; (b) Electron micrograph of purified CHIK-VLPs at 2, 00,000 X.

Chikungunya virus (CHIKV) has now emerged as one of the most important mosquito- transmitted arbovirus of public health significance. Vaccination is the most effective way of protecting humans and limiting further CHIKV transmission. Currently, there are no licensed antivirals and vaccines available commercially. Since 1960 various efforts have been made to develop a vaccine against the chikungunya virus. A number of strategies have been used for CHIKV vaccine development, including inactivated virus formulations, live-attenuated virus vaccines, DNA vaccines, chimeric virus vaccines, a recombinant adenovirus vaccine, subunit protein vaccines and a virus-like particle (VLP) formulation. Among all, some of the vaccine candidates have reached the preclinical stage in nonhuman primates (NHP) and first-level evaluation in humans (Ahola et al., 2015).

The Virus-Like particles (VLPs) are non-infectious, nanosized caged structures composed of viral structural proteins. The presence of complete structural proteins makes it an excellent antigen that strongly mimicks the native virus but lacks the viral genome, potentially yielding safer vaccine candidates. VLPs have the potency to elicit a protective response at lower doses of antigen, which significantly reduces vaccine cost (Noad & Roy, 2003). Recent studies have shown promising results in the development of CHIK-VLPs-based vaccines that developed in mammalian and baculovirus insect cell expression systems. These VLPs have been shown to elicit adequate neutralizing antibody responses in mice and non-human primates (Akhata et al., 2010; Metz et al., 2013).

Pichia pastoris has been shown to express a wide range of heterologous proteins either intracellular or in secreted form. In this study, CHIK-VLPs were expressed for the first time using the yeast (*P. pastoris*) expression system. *Pichia* cells readily grow in suspension cultures, which is a benefit of the yeast expression system. The *P. pastoris* yeast expression system used here offers several advantages for VLPs development: the techniques needed for molecular manipulation are simple, the ability to produce large-scale foreign proteins in their native conformation, operating costs are cheaper, simple chemical media and free from virus contamination, (Cregg et al., 2000; Vogl et al., 2013) makes it an attractive alternative platform.

For the development of CHIK-VLPs in *P. pastoris*, the full-length CHIKV structural polyprotein gene, C-E3-E2-6k-E1 was transformed into yeast *P. pastoris* under AOX1 promoter with the α-secretory signal of *Saccharomyces cerevisiae* . There are a limited number of vectors for *P. pastoris* but most of them are incorporated with tightly regulated and a very strong AOX promoter (Byrne, 2015; Cereghino et al., 2000). Here, the pPIC9K vector was used, which is known to generate multicopy integrants and for secreted expression of recombinant proteins using α-factor secretion signals. This α- factor secretion signal has a protease cleavage site that provides signals for secreted expression. The main advantage of expressing heterologous proteins in secreted form is that *P. pastoris* secretes a very small amount of native proteins therefore, the secreted heterologous protein mainly comprises the total protein content in the medium (Cereghino et al., 2000; Raemaekers et al., 1999).

In this study, recombinant *Pichia* clones have been generated with multicopy integrants, which harbor multiple copies of the structural polyprotein gene of CHIKV. These multicopy integrants were selected on the basis of their resistance to higher geneticin concentration, which correlates with the integration of multiple copies of the structural polyprotein gene of CHIKV. The product of the structural polyprotein gene is also separated from the secretory signal via host-specific endopeptidase resulting in the release of the fully processed structural polyprotein which assembled to form CHIK-VLPs (Cereghino et al., 2000; Cregg et al., 1993; Cregg et al., 2000).

In the case of *P. pastoris*, the transgene is integrated within the *Pichia* genome *via* homologous recombination at multiple sites, hence when the recombinant yeast is cultured and several times passaged; it is difficult to lose the target gene. Another advantage of selecting multicopy transformants is that if there is a mutation in one copy of the expression cassette, other copies resulting from the multiple integration processes may contribute markedly to the total amount of expressed protein rather than the mutant one (Cregg et al., 1993; Cregg et al., 2000).

The recombinant *Pichia* clones successfully having pPIC9K-CHIKV-C-E3-E2- 6K-E1 polyprotein expression cassette were expressing the proteins in soluble form. The expressed proteins were self-assembled into VLPs and released into the culture medium. Further, optimization of expression of CHIK-VLPs was done.

The optimized parameters were YPD with 2% methanol as induction medium and the yield of expressed protein was highest at 48 hrs post-induction. Induction of CHIK-VLPs expression was done using methanol which is very cheap and economical as a carbon source. In denaturing PAGE approximately 52 kDa, 35 kDa and 13 kDa bands have been observed that correspond to the approximate size of CHIKV E1/E2, capsid and E3 protein, respectively. So, these observations indicated the presence of all proteins for VLPs formation. These VLPs were successfully characterized by using different anti-CHIKV-specific antibodies *via* immunoblotting.

Our TEM results indicated that the VLPs were morphologically similar to the native CHIKV particles. The average diameter of Chikungunya cores was found approximately 40 nm which is consistent with the reported size of the chikungunya virus and other alphaviruses. Thus, this observation is in agreement with previous studies (Akhata et al., 2010; Metz et al., 2013).

CHAPTER 6

CHIK-VLP AS A DIAGNOSTIC TOOL

EVALUATION OF CHIK-VLPS AS A DIAGNOSTIC INTERMEDIATE IN SEROLOGICAL DIAGNOSIS

Chikungunya disease is associated with febrile illness and shares clinical signs with dengue and malaria. This often leads to misdiagnosis in the areas where these diseases are prevalent. Hence, a reliable and effective diagnostic method needs to be developed that should also be rapid and sensitive. Among the routine laboratory tests available for the diagnosis of CHIKV infection, virus isolation and plaque reduction neutralization test (PRNT) are used commonly for confirmation. However, these techniques have their own drawbacks of being time-consuming and tedious requiring more than a week for completion (Burke et al., 1982; Solomon et al., 1998).

In addition, the success of PRNT depends on the virus-specific neutralizing antibody titer which is generally not very high in Chikungunya infection.

In the absence of virus isolation and PRNT assay, a gene amplification method, particularly RT-PCR is the method of choice for early confirmatory diagnosis. However, some intrinsic limitations are always associated with the PCR-based detection techniques for example; the success of PCR-based methods greatly depends upon the viremic status of the patient.

It is difficult to detect viral RNA in the serum after defervescence or when the virus is eliminated after 5–7 days of onset of fever. Further virus isolation, PRNT, and RT-PCR are generally restricted to reference laboratories having highly trained technical manpower and resources. Furthermore, a high-precision instrument for amplification and detection of amplified products is also needed. Due to these intricacies, early diagnosis of infection demands a parallel method of choice that can be used to diagnose reliably CHIKV infection. Interestingly, the enzyme linked immunosorbent assay (ELISA) based methods also allow the confirmation of viral infections, even if the virus is removed completely by the immune system. ELISA-based diagnostic tests hold a great promise for the economic and convenient diagnosis of viral infections.

In this study, an indirect microplate IgM ELISA was standardized using the purified CHIK-VLPs, as antigens. VLPs-based IgM ELISA described in this study was specific for the detection of anti-CHIKV antibodies in human patient sera. In comparison with the E2 subunit antigen, the VLPs revealed higher sensitivity and specificity. It did not cross-react with clinical samples from symptomatically similar infections including Dengue and Japanese encephalitis. Furthermore, none of the apparently healthy samples showed any reactivity with the developed IgM-ELISA. These data suggest that CHIK- VLPs could be used for reliable and confirmatory diagnosis of Chikungunya infections.

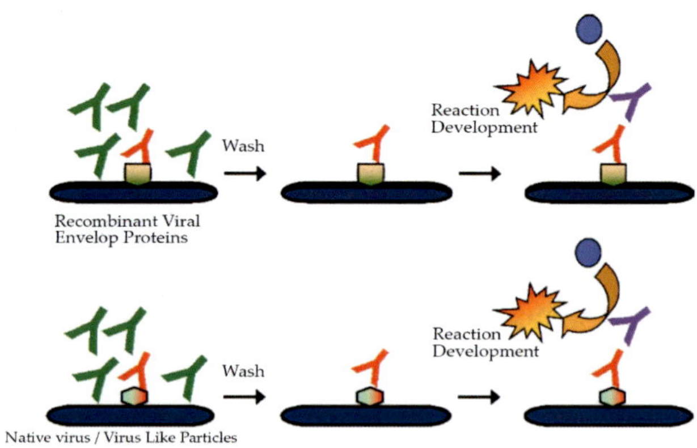

Figure 6.1: Representation of ELISA scheme. Principally in a normal ELISA format, the virus envelope protein can be replaced by Virus-Like particles (VLPs) that usually mimic the structure / morphologically and antigenicity of native CHIKV, suggesting that they have potential for use in chikungunya diagnosis.

Reactivity of CHIK-VLPs with Standard Anti-CHIKV Sera

The antigenicity of CHIK-VLPs was further confirmed using rabbit polyclonal serum raised against purified native CHIKV and recombinant E2-protein. The CHIK- VLPs used as antigen to coat microplates and their reactivity to anti-CHIKV native antigen sera and anti-CHIK-E2 specific serum was examined. Two-fold serial dilutions of rabbit serum starting from 1:100 dilution were subjected to the ELISA to detect antibodies. As depicted in Fig. 6.2, reactivity was observed up to 1:25600 ELISA titer with anti-CHIK- E2 specific serum and 1:51200 ELISA titer with anti-CHIKV native antigen serum, demonstrating that the VLPs possess antigenic similarity to that of native CHIKV and its subunit surface proteins like E2. It was concluded that the CHIK-VLPs can also be used as potential antigens for the detection of anti-CHIKV IgM antibodies in patients' sera.

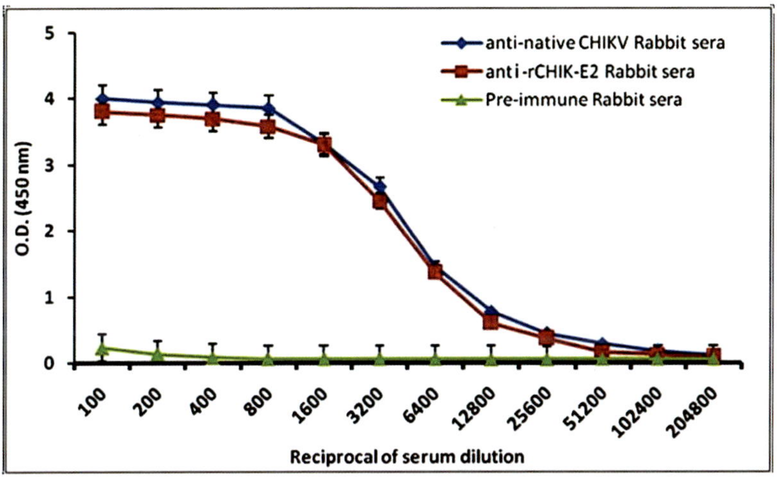

Figure 6.2: Antigenicity of CHIK-VLPs: Antigenic specificity of expressed CHIK-VLPs was determined by ELISA. Rabbit polyclonal sera were used to confirm shared antigenicity between CHIK-VLPs and native CHIKV antigen: anti-native CHIKV IgG responses and anti-rCHIK-E2 IgG responses were evaluated; Microplates were coated with purified VLPs (300 ng/well) and used to detect CHIKV-specific antibodies. Two-fold serially diluted rabbit sera starting from 1:100 was examined. Preimmune rabbit sera were included as the control.

Optimization of CHIK-VLPs for IgM ELISA

To determine the optimal concentration of yeast-derived CHIK-VLPs for detection of CHIKV IgM by indirect ELISA, the CHIK-VLPs were serially diluted from 10µg/ml to 1µg/ml. Confirmed positive and negative patient serum samples were then tested against different dilutions of CHIK-VLPs as antigens. The highest ratio of absorbance value for positive to negative serum was obtained using 3µg/ml of CHIK- VLPs (Fig. 6.2). This concentration of protein was therefore used in further experiments to evaluate the diagnostic potential for detection of CHIKV-specific IgM antibody. An indirect IgM microplate ELISA protocol was optimized using 300 ng of CHIK-VLPs. An optimal assay condition with a minimal background was established.

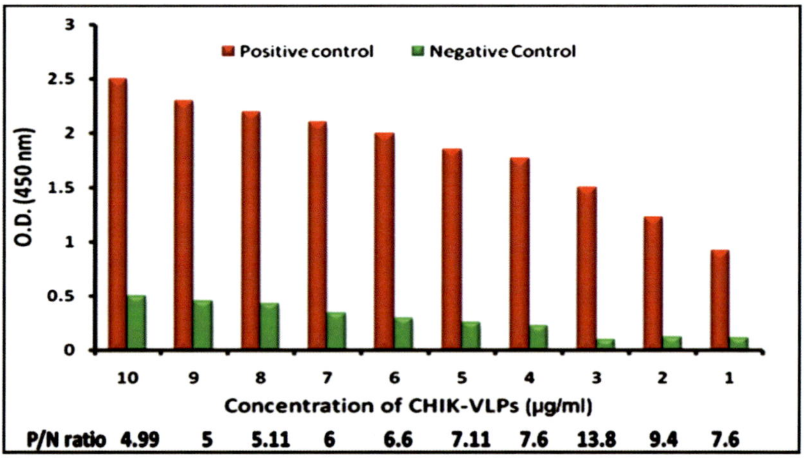

Figure 6.2: Optimization of CHIK-VLPs concentration for in-house IgM ELISA. ELISA plate was coated with different concentrations of antigens and evaluated for their reactivity with confirmed chikungunya positive or negative samples. Absorbance was read at 450 nm. The P/N ratio is the OD value of positive sera/OD value of negative sera at 450 nm.

COMPARATIVE EVALUATION OF CHIK-VLPS IGM MICROPLATE ELISA AND RCHIK-E2 IGM ELISA WITH NATIVE CHIKV IGM ELISA

For comparative analysis, an in-house purified native CHIKV antigen-based indirect IgM ELISA was considered as the reference standard. A panel of 100 human serum samples was initially screened by this native CHIKV IgM ELISA. This revealed 37 samples to be positive and 63 as negative for anti CHIKV IgM. Subsequently, all the samples were processed for detection of IgM antibodies by CHIK-VLPs and rCHIK-E2 protein-based IgM ELISA. A total of 36 and 34 samples were found positive for IgM antibodies by indirect ELISA employing CHIK-VLPs and rCHIK-E2 as antigens respectively. In all the ELISA formats, three standard positive and three standard negative samples were used. Figure 6.3 represents the mean values of standard positive and negative samples. The results with standard positive samples revealed mean O.D. ranging from 2.5 to 3.2 in all formats. Similarly, the standard negative samples revealed low mean O.D. ranging from 0.07 to 0.21 in all three formats. The mean absorbance of the standard positive samples was found to be significantly higher than the standard negative samples (P<0.0001) (Fig. 6.3).

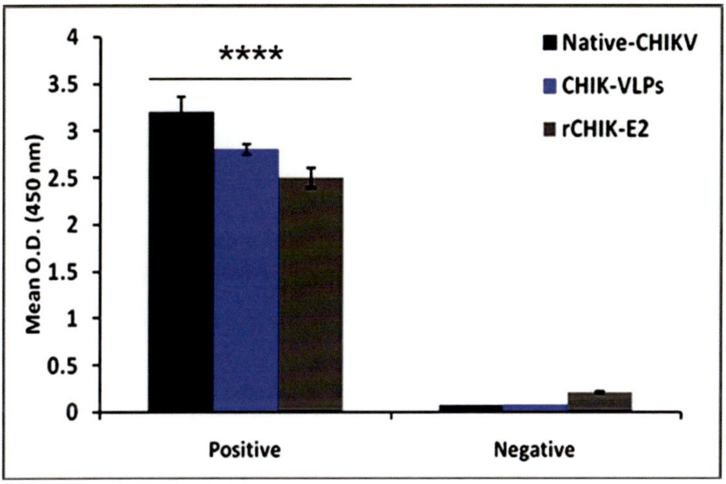

Figure 6.3: Mean OD values of the standard positive and standard negative samples used in the study.

Subsequently, the results of test samples revealed a mean O.D. ranging from 1.3 to 1.6 for the positive samples and 0.10 to 0.17 for negative samples in all the three formats (Fig. 6.4). The comparative evaluation of CHIK-VLPs and rCHIK-E2 based IgM ELISA revealed a significantly higher mean OD values in CHIK-VLPs based indirect ELISA format (P<0.0001).

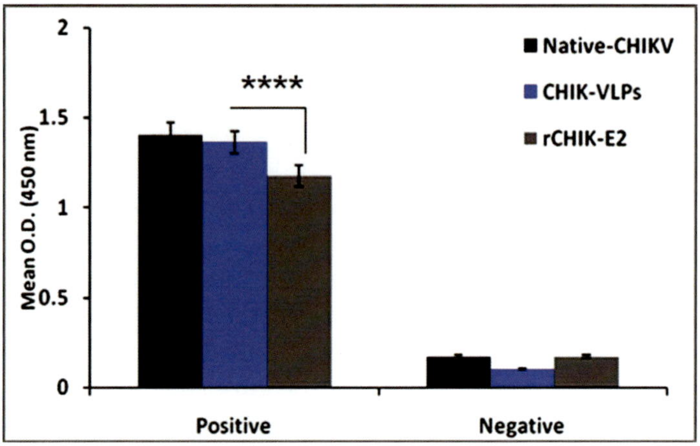

Figure 6.4: Mean OD values of the positive and negative samples used in the study.

Comparative O.D. values with different categories of sample panel are depicted in Fig. 6.5. The results with clinical samples in purified native CHIKV-based ELISA revealed higher O.D. values ranging from 0.65 to 3.15 in positive samples and 0.04 to 0.3 in negative samples (Fig. 6.5 a). Comparative evaluation with CHIK-VLPs based indirect IgM ELISA also revealed similar O.D. ranging from 0.63 to 2.92 compared to 0.06-0.35 in the case of negative samples (Fig. 6.5 b). The rCHIK-E2-based IgM ELISA revealed slightly lower O.D. ranging from 0.58 to 2.65 with positive samples; whereas the negative samples revealed an O.D. ranging from 0.08 to 0.42 (Fig. 6.5 c). None of the CHIKV antigens were found to be cross-reactive with serum samples from Dengue and Japanese encephalitis infected, and apparently healthy individuals (Fig. 6.5).

Comparative analysis of CHIK-VLPs and purified native CHIKV ELISA revealed a mismatch of just 3 samples. Out of these 3 samples, 2 were found positive in native CHIKV ELISA (Table 6.1). The comparison between purified native CHIKV and rCHIK-E2-based ELISA revealed a discordance result in 6 samples. Three out of these 6 samples were found positive by native CHIKV-based ELISA (Table 6.2) the sensitivity and specificity of CHIK-VLPs-based ELISA were found to be higher compared to E2-based ELISA. Further, PPV and NPV were also found better for CHIK-VLPs-based ELISA. These results indicate the superiority of CHIK-VLPs over rCHIK-E2-based ELISA in comparison to the in-house purified native CHIKV-based ELISA.

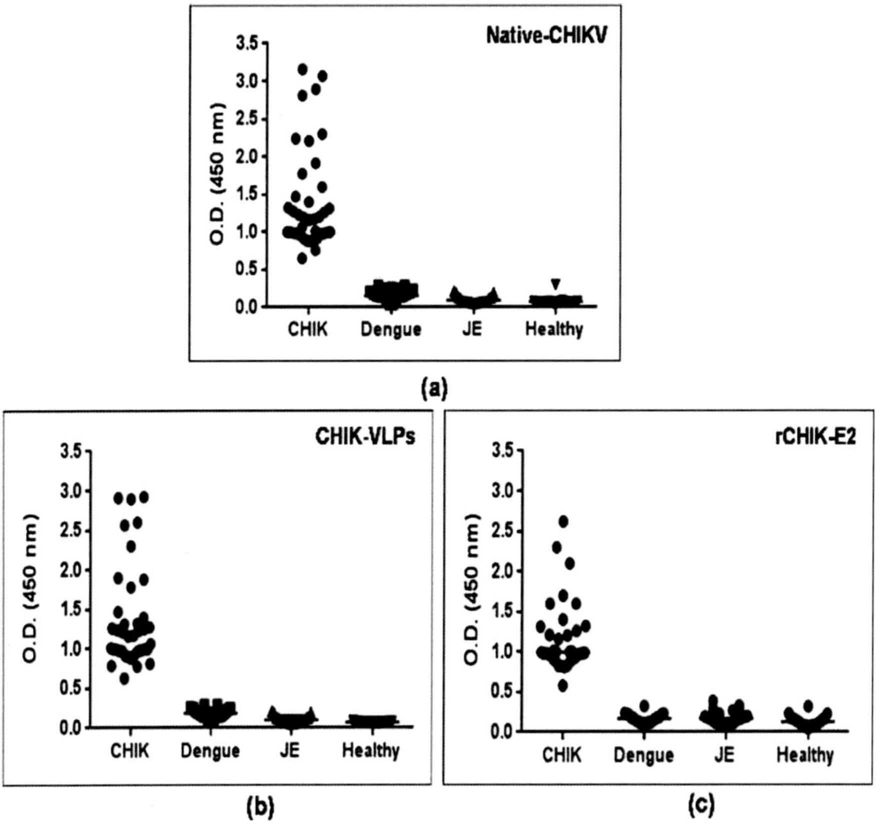

Figure 6.5: Evaluation of clinical samples with all ELISA formats; (a) Evaluation of CHIK-native based IgM ELISA on clinical samples; (b) Evaluation of CHIK-VLPs based IgM ELISA on clinical samples; (c) Evaluation of rCHIK-E2 based IgM ELISA on clinical samples; The O. D. profile of different kind of human patient samples (Dengue and Japanese encephalitis) including healthy controls as obtained through the IgM- ELISA specific to the different antigens (40 samples from the Chikungunya panel and 20 samples from others each panel). No cross-reactivity was obtained when different panels of the samples were analyzed by IgM ELISA specific to the CHIK-VLPs, rCHIKE2 and CHIK-native. The comparative analysis of the samples by CHIK-VLPs and native CHIKV revealed 97% concordance, while analysis of the samples by rCHIK-E2 and native CHIKV revealed 94% concordance (Table- 6.3). These data suggest that CHIK-VLPs could be used for reliable and confirmatory diagnosis of Chikungunya infections.

Table 6.1: Comparative analysis of a panel of serum samples analyzed by the CHIK- VLPs based indirect IgM ELISA and the Native-CHIKV based indirect IgM ELISA

Native-CHIKV-based IgM ELISA		Positive	Negative	Total
CHIK-VLPs	Positive	36	2	38
based IgM	Negative	1	61	62
ELISA	Total	37	63	100

Table 6.2: Comparative analysis of a panel of serum samples analyzed by the rCHIK-E2 based indirect IgM ELISA and the Native-CHIKV based indirect IgM ELIS

Native-CHIKV-based IgM ELISA		Positive	Negative	Total
rCHIK-E2	Positive	34	3	37
based IgM	Negative	3	60	63
ELISA	Total	37	63	100

Table 6.3: Comparative evaluation of CHIK-VLPs based indirect IgM ELISA and rCHIK-E2 based indirect IgM ELISA with respect to in-house native CHIKV-based IgM ELISA*

Agreement IgM ELISA	CHIK-VLPs based	rCHIK-E2 based IgM ELISA
A **Concordance %**	97	94
B **Sensitivity %**	97.29	91.89
C **Specificity %**	96.82	95.23
D **Positive predictive value (PPV) %**	94.73	91.89
E **Negative predictive value (NPV) %**	98.38	95.23

*Sucrose gradient purified native CHIKV based detection of specific IgM was considered as reference standard control. According to which 37 IgM positive 63 IgM negative samples were characterized.

[a] [(Number of samples positive by both methods + number of samples negative by both method)/(total number of samples)] × 100

[b] [True positive/(true positive + false negative)] × 100 [c] [True negative/(true negative + false positive)] × 100 [d] [True positive/(true positive + false positive)] × 100 [e] [True negative/(true negative + false negative)] × 100

As there is no licensed antiviral therapy or vaccine available for CHIKV, a specific detection system is the need of the hour. Several techniques for CHIKV detection including immunofluorescence technology, plaque assay and virus isolation have been reported. However, the complexity of these techniques has led to their replacement with more convenient methods e.g. RT-PCR and ELISA. RT-PCR is a highly specific and sensitive test for CHIKV but the reagents and equipment are too costly for its widespread use (Khan et al., 2014).

Though, virus isolation is considered as the gold standard. However, this is time-consuming, laborious and requires a BSL-3 facility. Therefore, it is not the method of choice and is of academic importance. The plaque reduction neutralization test (PRNT) is the standard method for confirmation and typing of a virus in which four-fold or greater increase in the virus-specific neutralizing antibody titer confirms the virus infection. However, the specific requirement of cell culture and virus handling facilities in the laboratory limit its routine use, in addition, it is time-consuming and tedious, requiring more than a week for completion. In contrast, ELISA-based assays are amenable to high throughput, low turnover time and remote field settings.

Detection of IgM antibodies of CHIKV in suspected patients is a useful tool for diagnosis as it can be detected as early as 4–5 days after the onset of fever and generally persists for several months. The earlier whole virus was being used as an antigen for detection of serum IgM but it was associated with biohazard risk. Handling of live viruses also requires a BSL3 laboratory and expertise. Hence, specific proteins produced by recombinant DNA technology (RDT) are now being widely used for CHIKV diagnostics instead of whole live viruses. Recombinant proteins are also economical compared to the production of native antigens in either cell cultures or suckling mice brains.

The success of serological assays inherently depends on the quality of the antigen. Replacement of cell culture-derived native CHIKV antigen by recombinant virus protein leads to improved specificity. However, the limitation includes compromised sensitivity, due to the availability of limited immunogenic epitopes. Since the subunit protein candidates are just a part of the native virus, a considerable amount of immunogenic epitopes are missed. The Virus-Like particles (VLPs) are non-infectious, nanosized caged structures composed of complete viral structural proteins. The presence of complete structural proteins makes it an excellent antigen that strongly mimics the native virus.

Currently, available commercial ELISA and ICT kits suffer from the issues of poor sensitivity and specificity and many products were withdrawn from the market (Prat et al., 2014). The VLPs-based diagnostic assay provides a promising alternative for the detection of CHIKV infection with a high degree of sensitivity and specificity. In this study, the potential application of CHIK-VLPs for clinical diagnosis of CHIKV was evaluated with acute phase human patient serum samples. Prior to evaluation with clinical sera, the CHIK-VLPs were first tested with their immunogenicity against hyper immune sera raised against both native virus and recombinant CHIKV immunogenic surface protein (E2). The high reactivity confirms the potential of CHIK-VLPs as an antigen molecule in indirect IgM ELISA format.

The comparative analysis of CHIK-VLPs based IgM ELISA with both standard purified native CHIKV and rCHIK-E2 based ELISA revealed that CHIK-VLPs are sensitive as well as specific in picking up CHIKV-specific IgM antibodies. CHIK-VLPs were found to be most effective in terms of recognizing the CHIKV-specific IgM from patients' sera with 97% concordance, 97.29% sensitivity and 96.82% specificity compared to the standard purified native CHIKV. Both sensitivity and specificity were also found to be higher compared to rCHIK-E2-based ELISA. Cross-reactivity was also not observed with dengue and JE patient sera and also with healthy human sera. Thus it is concluded that the present study for detection of Chikungunya IgM antibody by indirect ELISA using CHIK-VLPs as an antigen is specific, rapid and easy to perform and therefore can be a useful tool for rapid surveillance of CHIKV suspected samples. The most important advantage of this assay is that it can differentiate chikungunya infection from dengue fever, making it an extremely useful screening assay in many endemic areas where both dengue and chikungunya are co-circulating.

In conclusion, the overall comparable sensitivity and specificity of the CHIK- VLPs-based IgM-ELISA achieved in this study offers a promising economical tool for clinical diagnosis as well as rapid surveillance of CHIKV infection in endemic areas.

CHAPTER 7

CHIK-VLPS AS VACCINE CANDIDATES

EVALUATION OF THE IMMUNOGENIC POTENTIAL OF CHIK-VLPS IN BALB/C MICE

Vaccination is the most effective way of protecting humans and limiting further CHIKV transmission. Currently, there are no licensed antivirals or vaccines available commercially. Since 1960 various efforts have been made to develop a vaccine against CHIKV. A number of strategies have been used for CHIKV vaccine development, including inactivated virus formulations, live-attenuated virus vaccines, DNA vaccines, chimeric virus vaccines, a recombinant adenovirus vaccine, subunit protein vaccines and a virus-like particle (VLP) formulation. Among these, some of the vaccine candidates have reached the preclinical stage in nonhuman primates (NHP) and first-level evaluation in humans (Ahola et al., 2015).

Conventional inactivated and live attenuated vaccines have been shown to be immunogenic in humans. However, the requirement of a large quantity of CHIKV and BSL3 containment for vaccine manufacturing are the main hurdles. Although live-attenuated vaccines elicit an effective balanced immune response, but associated with the risk of reversion to virulence (Noad et al., 2003). A live-attenuated CHIKV vaccine (TSI-GSD- 218), showed promising results in phase I (McClain et al., 1998) and phase II (Edelman et al., 2000) clinical trials, its further development was discontinued because some side effects like arthralgia were seen in 8% of volunteers (Hoke et al., 2012). DNA vaccines having C–E2–E1 construct were found to generate neutralizing antibodies in mice and nonhuman primates but they required more than five immunizations. Thus, it was ineffective in generating antibody responses in humans (Ahola et al., 2015).

The Virus-Like particles (VLPs) are non-infectious, nanosized caged structures composed of viral structural proteins. The presence of complete structural proteins makes it an excellent antigen that strongly mimics the native virus but lacks the viral genome, potentially yielding safer vaccine candidates. VLP-based vaccines induced an effective immune response at lower doses of antigen, which significantly reduces vaccine cost (Noad & Roy, 2003). Earlier studies have shown promising results in the development of CHIK-VLPs-based vaccines that developed in mammalian and baculovirus insect cell expression systems. These VLPs have been shown to elicit an adequate neutralizing antibody response in mice and non-human primates (Akhata et al., 2010; Metz et al., 2013).

But these VLPs have some disadvantages; CHIK-VLPs based on mammalian cell expression systems are related to higher production cost and lower controllability and productivities. Moreover, in the baculovirus insect cell expression system, co-production of enveloped baculovirus particles contaminates the vaccine candidate. Because adjuvant activity has also been shown to be associated with baculovirus, if a vaccine is not free from them baculovirus particles may develop immunogenicity (Hervas-Stubbs et al., 2007). Moreover, baculovirus particles and VLPs are difficult to separate; VLPs produced in this system have to undergo either chemical inactivation treatments or several downstream processing steps to eliminate baculovirus infectivity that may impair the quality of the VLP and also increases the production cost (Rueda et al., 2000).

Pichia cells are readily adaptable to grow in suspension cultures, which is a key benefit of the yeast expression system. The *Pichia pastoris* (*P. pastoris*) yeast expression system used in this study confers several advantages for VLPs development: the simplicity of the techniques needed for molecular manipulation, the ability to produce large-scale foreign proteins in their native conformation, cheaper operating costs, simple defined chemical media and free from virus contamination (Vogl et al., 2013). It offers an attractive alternative platform to current mammalian or insect cell culture processes. Furthermore, yeast-expressed VLPs vaccines (e.g. hepatitis B virus VLPs and human papillomavirus VLPs) have been proven to be safe and effective (Roldão et al., 2010). The first yeast-derived

VLP vaccine (Hepatitis B virus VLP vaccine) (Recombivax HB® Merck and Co., USA) received FDA approval in 1986. To date, a handful of *P. Pastoris* -derived VLP-based vaccines have been approved by US FDA and are commercially available worldwide against the hepatitis B virus. In India, Enivac HB (Panacea Biotec Ltd.), Revac-B+™ (Bharat Biotech International Ltd.), Shanvac™-B (Shantha Biotechnics Ltd.) are the commercially available VLPs-based vaccines against hBsAg that derives from *P. pastoris* (Antonio et al., 2010). Other *P. pastoris*-derived Dengue VLPs (Mani et al. 2013), HPV-16 VLPs (Bazan et al., 2009) and Norovirus VLPs (Xia et al., 2007) are shown to elicit good neutralizing antibody titer.

With these advantages, we first time exploited the *P. pastoris* expression system to develop a CHIK-VLPs-based vaccine candidate and evaluated both humoral and cellular responses in the mouse model.

Determination of Humoral Immune Response

ELISA Antibody Titer (Total IgG titer)

To assay the antibody response in post-vaccinated mice sera following immunization, an indirect ELISA using CHIK-VLPs was performed from the pooled sera samples collected from individual mice at 14, 28, 42, 56 and 140 days of post-vaccination. The highest IgG endpoint titer to CHIK-VLPs was 4×10^3 in sera of 40μg CHIK-VLPs group whereas it was 2×10^3 in 20μg CHIK-VLPs and 1×10^3 in the 10μg CHIK-VLPs group at 14 days post-immunization.

The highest IgG endpoint titer after the first booster (28 days) was 1.6×10^4 in the 40μg CHIK-VLPs group whereas it was 4×10^3 in 20μg CHIK-VLPs and only 2×10^3 in 10μg CHIK-VLPs groups. The peak ELISA antibody titer was obtained 42 days post-vaccination After the second booster (42 days), antibody titers were 3.2×10^4, 2.56×10^4 and 8×10^3 in mice immunized with 40μg, 20μg and 10μg CHIK-VLPs respectively. Serum anti- CHIK-VLPs antibody levels in the mice immunized with all three concentrations were significantly higher than controls on the 42nd day ($^{\#}P < 0.0001$) whereas on 56 and 140 days was significantly higher in 40μg and 20μg concentration with respect to control mice sera ($^{\#}P < 0.0001$) and the same pattern was found up to 140 days post-vaccination. Serum antibody titer induced by CHIK-VLPs increased in a dose-dependent manner. Following booster immunization, ELISA titers substantially increased. The antibody titer in 40μg CHIK-VLPs was found to be significantly higher than

20μg CHIK-VLPs (****P< 0.0001) and 10μg CHIK-VLPs ($^{\$}$p< 0.0001) (Fig.7.1).

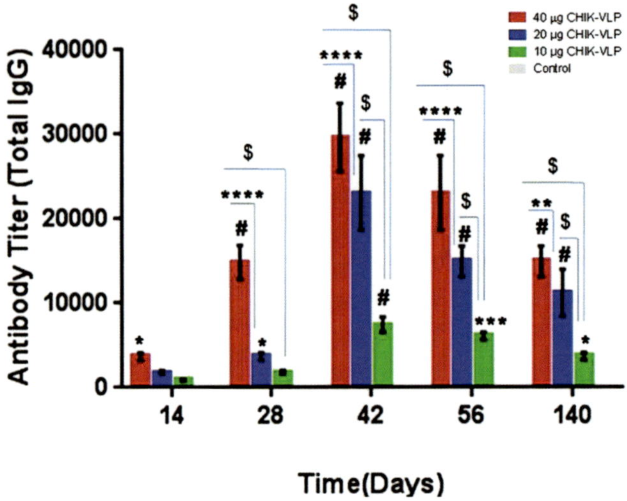

Figure 7.1: Measurement of serum IgG antibody titers in immunized Balb/c mice. Sera collected after the first booster 14, 28, 42, 56 and 140 days of post-vaccination from immunized groups with 40μg CHIK-VLPs, 20μg CHIK-VLPs and 10μg CHIK-VLPs and antibody titer was measured by indirect ELISA. Data represented in mean antibody titers with SD of ten Balb/C mice in each group. Analysis was done by one-way ANOVA (Fisher LSD Method). ****P<0.0001(significance with respect to 20μg CHIK-VLPs);

$^{\$}$P< 0.0001; (significance with respect to 10μg CHIK-VLPs); $^{\#}$P< 0.0001; ***P< 0.001;

*P< 0.01 (significance with respect to control).

IGG SUBTYPING DEMONSTRATES HIGH LEVELS OF IGG1 AND IGG2A

Due to the strong antibody response, isotyping analysis was performed from the pooled sera samples collected seven days after the second booster to determine the predominant isotypes of antibodies produced in mice in response to vaccination. The cut- off value for the assays was calculated as the mean OD (+2 SD) from sera of the control group assayed at 1:1000 dilutions. Significantly (#p< 0.0001) elevated levels of all four isotypes IgG1, IgG2a, IgG2b and IgG3 were observed in all three groups (40μg

CHIK- VLPs, 20μg CHIK-VLPs and 10μg CHIK-VLPs) compared to control group. Among the IgG subclasses, IgG1 and IgG2a appeared to have the highest and approximately the same levels, although IgG3 levels were also high while IgG2b levels were the lowest. Immunization of different doses of CHIK-VLPs with FCA showed a balanced immune response with the approximately high and same amount of IgG1 and IgG2a. No significant difference has been seen between the level of IgG1 and IgG2a, whereas with respect to IgG2b the level of IgG1 and IgG2a were found to be significantly higher ($P< 0.0001). The level of IgG3 was found to be significantly lower (¤P< 0.0001) than IgG1 and IgG2a in all doses of CHIK-VLPs (Fig.7.2).

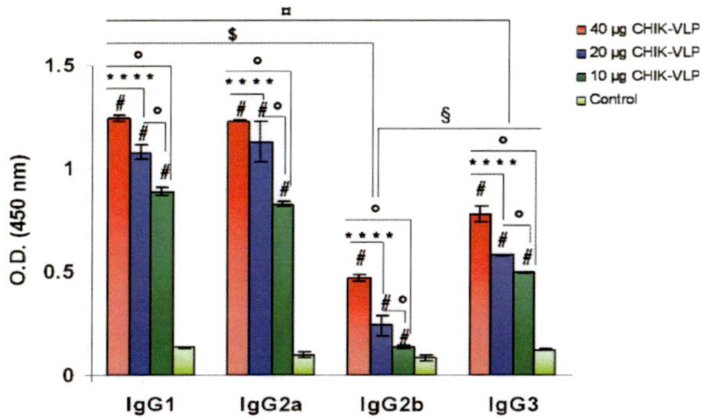

Figure 7.2: Measurement of serum IgG isotypes titers in immunized BALB/c mice. Profile of IgG isotypes in sera from immunized animal groups (40μg CHIK-VLPs, 20μg CHIK-VLPs and 10μg CHIK-VLPs). Data represented as mean antibody titers with SD of ten Balb/C mice in each group Analysis was done by one-way ANOVA, (Fisher LSD) #P< 0.0001(significance with to control); ****P< 0.0001(significance with respect to 20μg CHIK-VLPs); °P< 0.0001(significance with respect to 10μg CHIK-VLPs); $P< 0.0001(significance with respect to IgG2b); §P< 0.001(significance with respect to IgG2b); ¤P< 0.0001(significance with respect to IgG3).

YEAST DERIVED CHIK-VLPS GENERATED A HIGH TITER OF NEUTRALIZING ANTIBODIES THAT RECOGNIZED NATIVE CHIKV

To evaluate whether anti-CHIK-VLPs are able to recognize native Chikungunya virus or not, an immunofluorescence assay and indirect ELISA were performed. 1st and 2nd booster sera raised against 40 μg CHIK-VLPs were analyzed by Immunofluorescence in CHIKV-infected Vero cells. Both booster sera samples containing antibodies were found highly specific and sensitive to recognizing CHIKV in infected cells (Fig. 7.3 a). A higher level of CHIKV antigen was detected by anti-CHIK-VLPs of the 2nd booster compared to the 1st booster. The sera of mock immunized mice did not show any fluorescence. Thus, mice sera of both the boosters of different groups were found to recognize the native chikungunya virus with a high endpoint titer. A dose-dependent antibody titer has been seen with a significant difference in antibody titer of all three doses of both boosters (****P< 0.0001) (Fig. 7.3 b)

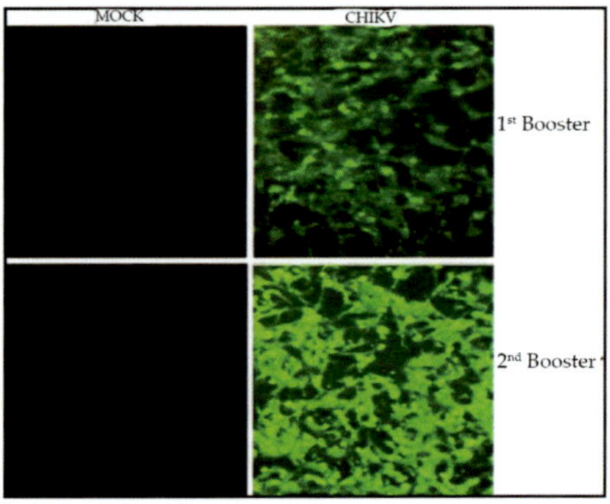

(A)

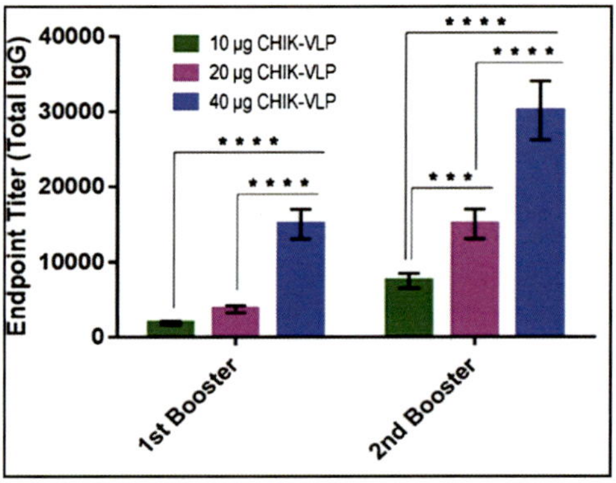

(B)

Figure 7.3: Antibody raised against CHIK-VLPs were evaluated for their specificity against Chikungunya virus. (A) Determination of immunofluorescence against Chikungunya virus by using sera of different boosters of 40µg CHIK-VLPs ; (B) Antibody titration of both boosters of all groups against Chikungunya. Data represented as mean antibody titers with SD of ten Balb/C mice in each group Analysis was done by one-way ANOVA, (Fisher LSD) ****P< 0.0001.

IN VITRO VIRUS NEUTRALIZATION ACTIVITY OF MICE SERA IMMUNIZED WITH CHIK- VLPS

The $PRNT_{50}$ titer of mice sera were 1:2048, 1:512 and 1:168 for 40µg CHIK-VLPs, 20µg CHIK-VLPs and 10µg CHIK-VLPs respectively (Fig. 7.4 a). This neutralization was further confirmed by using an Immunofluorescence assay. As seen in Fig. 7.4 b as compared to virus control reduction in fluorescence was achieved in 1:1024 dilution of mice sera immunized with 40µg CHIK-VLPs. These data support that antibodies raised against CHIK-VLPs were highly specific and recognize native CHIKV and mainly bind to CHIKV antigen on neutralization.

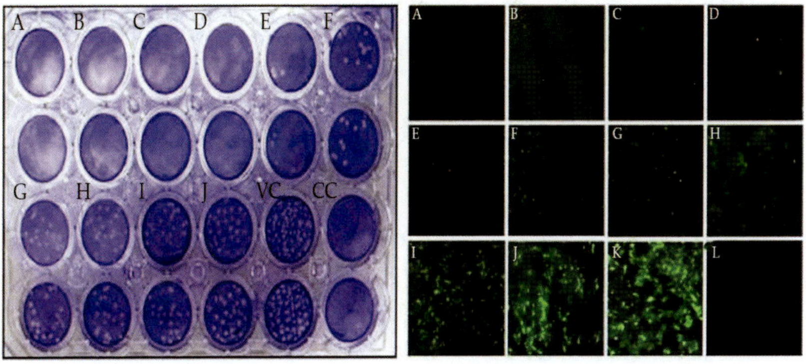

(A) Plaque reduction neutralization test (B) Fluorescent Microscopy

Figure 7.4: *In vitro* virus neutralization activity of mice sera immunized with CHIK- VLPs. (A) Titration of Chikungunya virus by plaque reduction neutralization test where mice sera are serially 2-fold diluted with 10^2 pfu CHIKV; A-J serial two-fold dilution of mice sera starting from 1:8 dilution to 1:4196 dilution and neutralize with 10^2 pfu Chikungunya virus, VC-Virus control, CC-cell control; (B) Detection of *in-vitro* neutralization of Chikungunya virus by IFT using anti-CHIKVE2 antibody at 10x; A-J serial two-fold dilution of mice sera starting from 1:8 dilution to 1:4196 dilution that neutralize 10^2 pfu Chikungunya virus; K-Virus control; L-Cell control.

IMMUNIZED MICE SHOWED FULL PROTECTION AND SURVIVAL FROM CHIKV

To evaluate the protective efficacy of CHIK-VLPs, *in vivo* neutralization was done in the suckling mouse model. It was observed that antibodies raised against CHIK-VLPs were neutralizing CHIKV significantly (**$p<0.001$).

Clinical symptoms associated with Chikungunya in mice like hind limb paralysis and retarded growth were not discernable in the CHIK-VLPs IgG treated mice group. Whereas, the mice that received control IgG and were infected with CHIKV exhibited the clinical symptoms at 4-7 days post-infection. All the mice from CHIKV infected group died in up to 7 days of post-infection, whereas all mice from the treated group survived and were healthy (Fig. 7.5 a). The body weight of mice, which had received passive immunization was similar to mock-infected mice, but showed significantly higher body weight gain compared to CHIKV-infected mice (***p<0.0001) (Fig. 7.5 b). Serum viremia was found to be 10-fold lower at day 3 dpi in IgG treat groups compared to CHIKV infected group (*p<0.01). At day 6 dpi, CHIKV RNA copies were found to be 2500 fold lower in treated groups compared to the CHIKV infected group (**p<0.001) (Fig. 7.5 c).

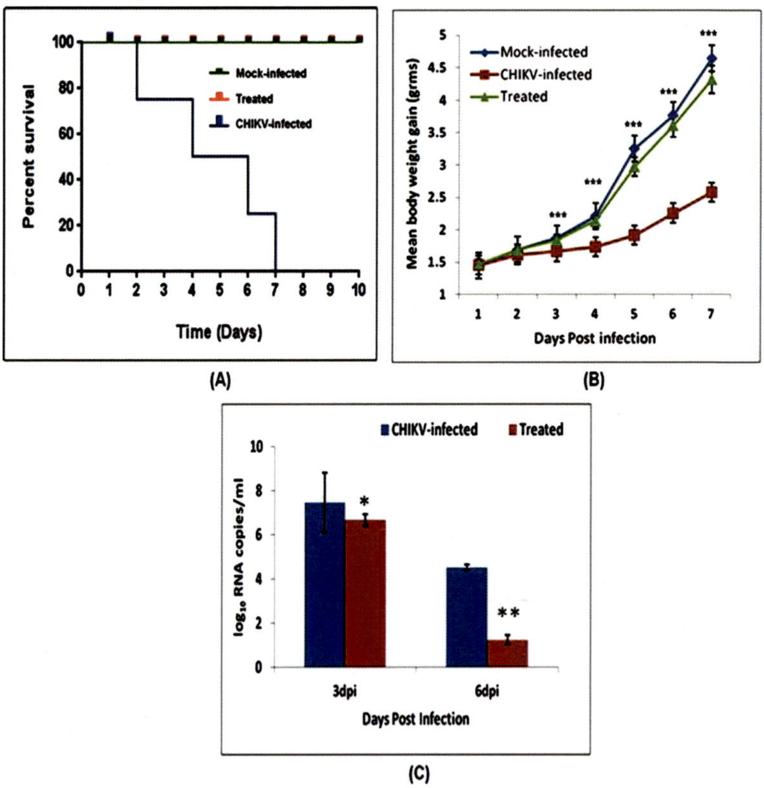

Figure 7.5: *In vivo* virus neutralization activity of mice sera immunized with CHIK- VLPs. (A) Percentage survival of all the mice groups. CHIKV-infected mice showed 100% mortality whereas treated mice that received CHIK-VLPs IgG and then infected with CHIKV showed a 100% survival rate same as mock-

infected mice that were neither infected with CHIKV nor received specific IgG; (B) Body weight gain measured on 1-7 day of post-infection. The treated mice group showed significantly higher (***p<0.0001) body weight gain than CHIKV infected mice group; (C) Serum viremia at 3dpi and 6 dpi. Serum viremia was found to be 10-fold lower at day 3dpi in IgG treated groups compared to the CHIKV infected group (*p<0.01). At day 6 dpi, 2500 fold lower CHIKV RNA copies were detected in treated groups compared to the CHIKV infected group (**p<0.001).

CELL-MEDIATED IMMUNE RESPONSE ELICITED BY CHIK-VLPS

Balance Th1/Th2 Response has been observed by Cytokine Profiling

Cytokine profiles of all immunized animal groups were studied by estimating the levels of IL-2, IL-4, IL-10, IFN-γ and TNF-α in the supernatants of splenocytes stimulated with different doses of CHIK-VLPs as antigens using sandwich ELISA. The expression levels of cytokines were determined with the help of a standard curve (Fig. 7.5) and presented as picograms per milliliter (pg/ml). A significant difference (****p< 0.0001) was observed in the expression levels of TNF-α and IL-10 whereas, IL-2, IL-4 and IFN-γ were significantly higher (***p< 0.005) in all the immunized animal groups compared to the control group.

In the case of IL-2 (Fig. 7.5), a significant difference (***P< 0.005) was observed among all the groups (40 μg CHIK-VLPs, 20 μg CHIK-VLPs and 10 μg CHIK- VLPs) compared to 72 hrs and 48 hrs. The expression level in 40 μg CHIK-VLPs was significantly high (****P< 0.0001 and $^{\square}$P< 0.0001) compared with 20 μg CHIK-VLPs and 10 μg CHIK-VLPs respectively at both the time points (72 hrs and 48 hrs) whereas, a significant difference ($^{\square}$P< 0.0001 and *P< 0.01) has been observed in the expression of 20 μg CHIK-VLPs in comparison to 10 μg CHIK-VLPs at 72 hrs and 48 hrs respectively. With respect to the control group, significance ($^{\#}$P< 0.0001) was observed in 40 μg CHIK- VLPs and 20 μg CHIK-VLPs at72 hrs and even at 40 μg CHIK-VLPs in 48 hrs. However, 10 μg CHIK-VLPs at72 hrs and 20 μg CHIK-VLPs at 48 hrs were found to significantly high (**P< 0.001) with respect to the control.

In the case of TNF-α (Fig. 7.5 b), a significant difference (***P< 0.005) was observed among all the groups (40 μg CHIK-VLPs, 20 μg CHIK-VLPs and 10 µg CHIK- VLPs) in comparison with 72hrs and 48 hrs. A dose-dependent pattern was seen.

The expression level of 40 µg CHIK-VLPs was significantly high (****P< 0.0001 and ¤P< 0.0001) in comparison with 20 µg CHIK-VLPs and 10 µg CHIK-VLPs respectively at both the time points (72 hrs and 48 hrs) whereas, a significant difference (**P< 0.001) has been observed in the expression of 20 µg CHIK-VLPs in comparison to 10 µg CHIK- VLPs at 72hrs; while, no difference has been observed in the expression level of 20 µg CHIK-VLPs and 10 µg CHIK-VLPs at 48 hrs. With respect to the control group, significance (#P< 0.0001) was observed in all groups at 72 hrs and even in 40 µg CHIK- VLPs at 48 hrs. Whereas, (**P< 0.001 and *P< 0.01) significance has been observed in 20 µg CHIK-VLPs and 10 µg CHIK-VLPs at 48 hrs with respect to the control.

In the case of IFN-γ (Fig. 7.5c), a significant difference (***P< 0.005) was observed among all the groups at 72 hrs and 48 hrs. The expression level of 40 µg CHIK-VLPs was significantly high (****P< 0.0001 and ¤P< 0.0001) in comparison with 20 µg CHIK-VLPs and 10 µg CHIK-VLPs respectively at both the time points (72 hrs and 48 hrs) whereas, a significance difference (¤P< 0.0001) was observed in the expression of 20 µg CHIK-VLPs in comparison to 10 µg CHIK-VLPs at 72 hrs and even at 48 hrs. With respect to the control group significance (#P< 0.0001) was observed in the entire VLPs immunized group at 72 hrs and even in 40 µg CHIK-VLPs and 20 µg CHIK- VLPs at 48 hrs. However, the expression of 10 µg CHIK-VLPs in 48 hrs was found to be significantly (**P< 0.001) high with respect to the control. In the case of IL-4 (Fig. 7.6), a significant difference (***P< 0.005) was observed among all the groups in comparison with 72 hrs and 48 hrs. The expression level of 40 µg CHIK-VLPs was significantly high (****P< 0.0001 and **P< 0.001) in comparison with 20 µg CHIK-VLPs at 72 hrs and 48 hrs respectively, whereas, a significant difference (¤P< 0.0001) has been observed in the expression of 40 µg CHIK-VLPs with respect to 10 µg CHIK-VLPs at both time points. However, a significant difference (*P< 0.01) has been observed in the expression of 20 µg CHIK-VLPs in comparison to 10 µg CHIK-VLPs at 72 hrs and even at 48 hrs. With respect to the control group, significance (#P< 0.0001) was observed in 40 µg CHIK-VLPs at both time points, whereas, the expression level of 20 µg CHIK-VLPs immunized group was (***P< 0.005 and **P< 0.001) significantly higher at 72 hrs and 48 hrs respectively with the control group. However, the expression of 10 µg CHIK-VLPs at 72 hrs was found to be significantly (*P< 0.01) high with respect to control, while no significance has been observed at 48 hrs compared to the control group.

In the case of IL-10 (Fig. 7.6b), a significant difference (****P< 0.0001) was observed among all the groups in comparison with 72hrs and 48 hrs. The expression level of 40 μg CHIK-VLPs was significantly high (****P< 0.0001 and $^{\square}$P< 0.0001) in comparison with 20 μg CHIK-VLPs and 10 μg CHIK-VLPs, respectively at both the time points, whereas, a significant difference ($^{\square}$P< 0.0001) has been observed in the expression of 20 μg CHIK-VLPs in comparison to 10 μg CHIK- VLPs at 72 hrs. No significance has been achieved at 20 μg CHIK- VLPs and 10 μg CHIK-VLPs at 48 hrs. With respect to the control group significance ($^{\#}$P< 0.0001) was observed among all groups at 72 hrs and even in 40 μg CHIK-VLPs at 48 hrs. Whereas, significance (**P< 0.001 and *P< 0.01) has been observed in 20 μg CHIK-VLPs and 10 μg CHIK-VLPs at 48 hrs with respect to control. Splenocytes from all groups responded to ConA non-specifically. The relative expression level of cytokines (IL-2, IL-4, IL-10, IFN-γ and TNF-α) in the immunized animal groups have been listed in Table 4.4 IL-2, TNF-α and IFN-γ mediate Th1 response and IL-4 and IL-10 mediate Th2 response. So here, we found higher expression of TNF-α, IL-10 and moderate expression of IL-2, IL-4 and IFN- γ which resulted in a balanced Th1/Th2 response.

Table 4.4: Expression level of cytokines in control (PBS immunized) and vaccinated (CHIK-VLPs immunized) animal groups

S.No.	Groups	IL-2 (pg/ml)	TNF-α (pg/ml)	IFN-γ (pg/ml)	IL-4 (pg/ml)	IL-10 (pg/ml)
1.	40 μg	211.28±10.5	1067.44±70.4	394.11±17.6	55.96±7.9	772.71±18.3
	CHIK-	5	4	5	4	0
	VLPs					
2.	20 μg	171.25±7.76	379.13±47.56	197.31±15.2	26.42±2.2	304.40±15.7
	CHIK-			7	3	7
	VLPs					
3.	10 μg	75.74±7.97	261.10±18.46	94.12±2.00	16.22±1.5	128.87±4.58
	CHIK-				2	
	VLPs					
4.	Control	14.89±3.31	24.69±9.08	8.37±0.02	6.18±2.20	4.58±0.19

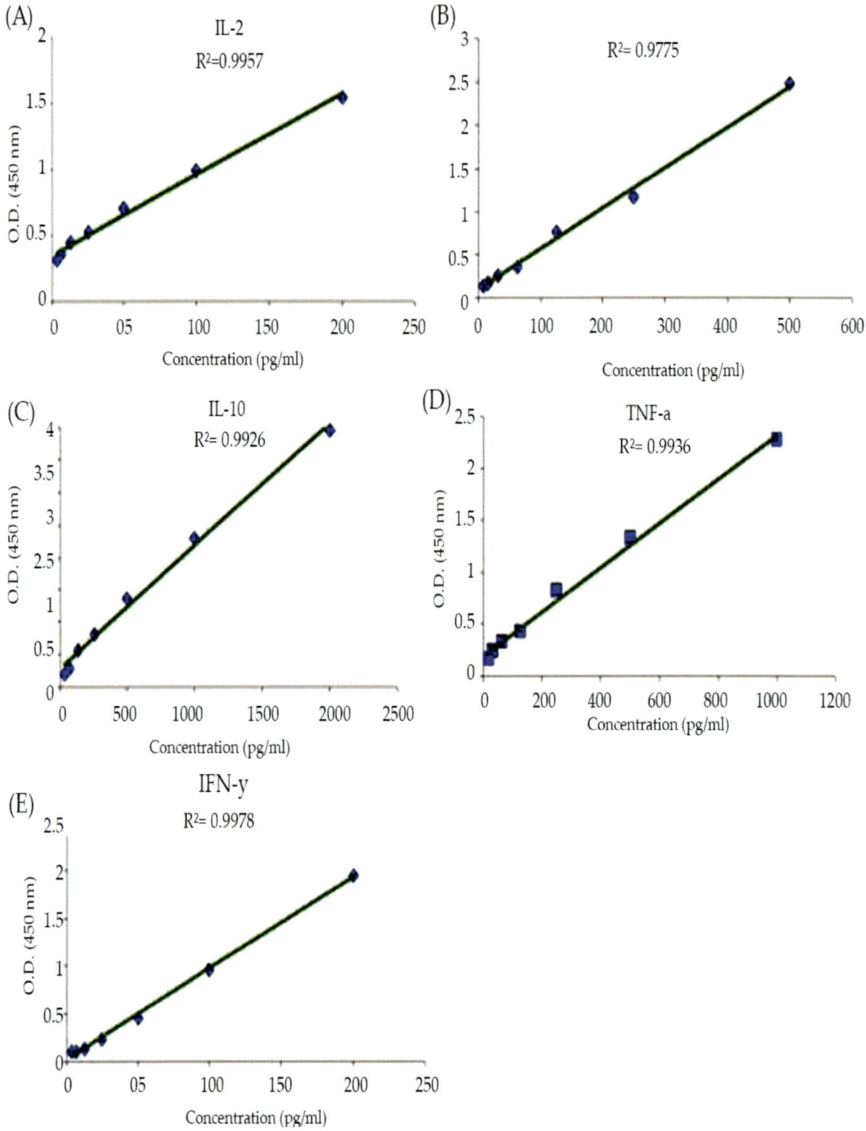

Figure 7.5: Cytokine standard curve. Recombinant cytokines were serially diluted and standard curves were generated for IL-2 (A); IL-4 (B); IL-10 (C); TNF-α (D) and IFN-γ (E) for estimating the levels of particular cytokine from the culture supernatant.

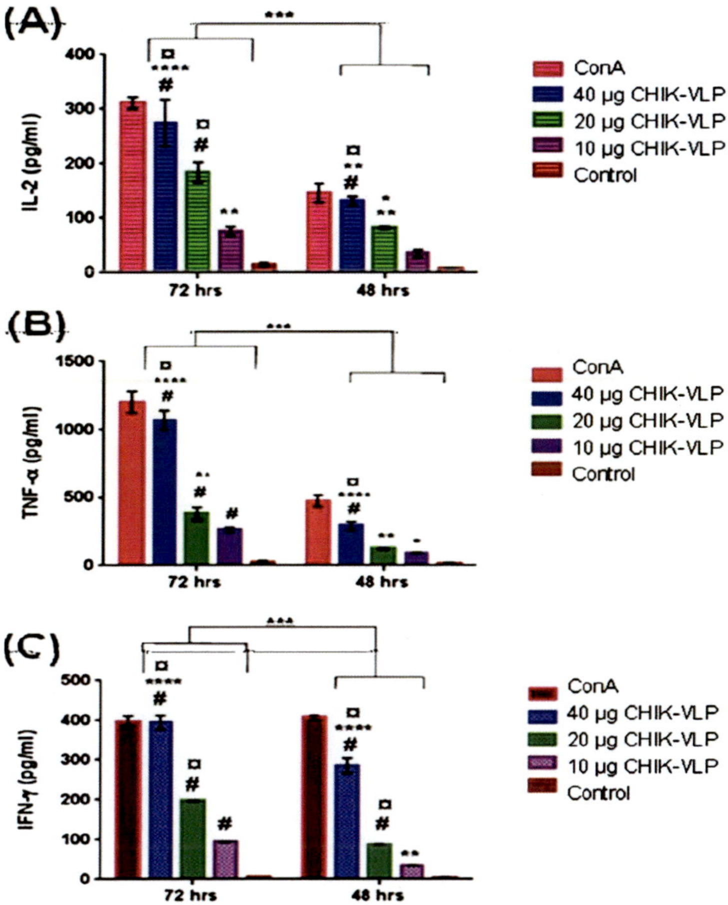

Figure 7.6: Measurement of Th1 cytokines expressed in the splenocytes of immunized mice groups. Graphs showing concentrations of IL-2 (A); TNF-α (B); IFN-γ (C) in picograms per milliliter (pg/ml). Each bar represents the average of 10 mice/group ± S.D and is representative of three independent experiments. Analysis was done by one-way ANOVA, (Fisher LSD Method). *P< 0.01; **P< 0.001; ***P< 0.005; ****P< 0.0001; #P< 0.0001; ¤P< 0.0001.

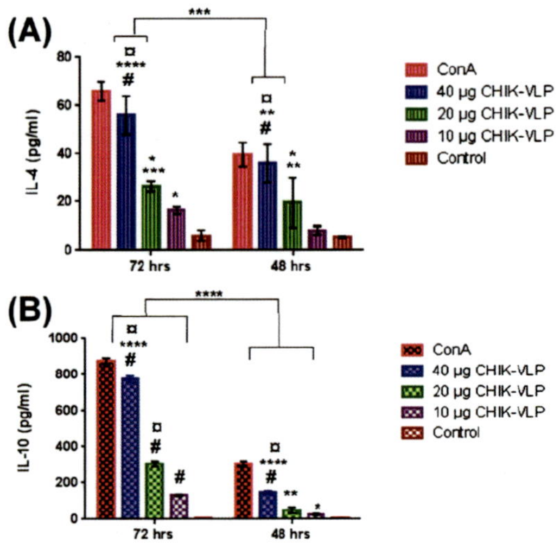

Figure 7.7: Measurement of Th2 cytokines expressed in the splenocytes of immunized mice groups. Graphs showing concentrations of IL-4 (A) and IL-10 (B) in picograms per milliliter (pg/ml). Each bar represents the average of 10 mice/group ± S.D and is representative of three independent experiments. Analysis was done by one-way ANOVA, (Fisher LSD Method). *P< 0.01; **P< 0.001; ***P< 0.005; ****P< 0.0001; #P< 0.0001;¤P< 0.0001.

The continuous expansion of CHIKV and increase in human morbidity make it one of the most important emerging arboviruses. There is a demand to develop a safe and effective CHIKV vaccine to protect humans and also to stop CHIKV transmission. Several strategies have been designed to combat CHIKV infections but none of these have been licensed yet and are not easily amenable to scale up.

VLPs have been known to stimulate similar immune responses as native viruses. Polyvalence of VLPs leads to a high frequency of crosslinking between B-cell receptors and VLPs epitopes that resulted in stronger humoral response as well as broader protection (Schwarz & Douglas, 2015). *Pichia pastoris* VLPs vaccines (e.g. hepatitis B virus VLPs and human papillomavirus VLPs) are commercially available. These VLPs have been administered as polyvalent antigens and have shown to elicit prophylactic activity and also have been proven to be safe and effective for human beings (Roldao et al., 2010; Grgacic & Anderson, 2006; Leroux-Roels et al., 2015). Therefore, the *Pichia* system proved economical for large-scale production of recombinant proteins (Byrne, 2015), so considering the safety and also the economic potential of the *Pichia* expression platform, our results indicate that *P. pastoris* can be an alternative host for large-scale and rapid production of Chikungunya VLPs.

VLPs stimulate innate as well as adaptive immune responses and act as safer effective vaccine candidates. Recently, a phase I clinical trial on CHIK-VLPs has been conducted by the National Institute of Health (NIH) and CHIK-VLPs have been shown to be safe, well-tolerated and immunogenic in human volunteers (Chang et al., 2014).

Our evaluation indicated that the CHIK-VLPs elicited both humoral and cell-mediated immune responses in mice. The humoral response was characterized by high titers of ELISA antibodies as well as high neutralizing titers by plaque reduction neutralization assay. All doses exhibited promising antibody titers. The peak ELISA antibody titer was obtained on the 42nd day post-vaccination; antibody titers were 3.2×10^4, 2.56×10^4 and 8×10^3 with 40μg, 20μg and 10μg CHIK-VLPs respectively. Humoral response plays a crucial role in neutralizing the viruses and their clearance. In the present study, antibodies raised against different doses of CHIK-VLPs were found to interact with native CHIKV, using anti-CHIK-VLPs sera in infected Vero cells. After demonstrating the successful recognition of native CHIKV, the virus neutralizing titer was determined for sera raised against different doses of CHIK-VLPs. The $PRNT_{50}$ titer of mice sera were 1:2048, 1:512 and 1:168 for 40μg, 20μg and 10μg CHIK-VLPs respectively.

In vivo neutralization assay was accomplished in suckling mice. It was observed that a substantial titer of CHIKV leads to the development of typical symptoms of Chikungunya that was confirmed by increased viremia, retarded growth and clinical symptoms like hind limb paralysis. Suckling mice were found to be protected as there was a-10 fold lower CHKV RNA copies at day 3 dpi and further 2500-fold lower CHIKV RNA copies were detected at day 6 dpi in IgG treated groups compared to the virus control group. Hence, it was concluded that the post-vaccinated sera of mice immunized with CHIK-VLPs were not only able to recognize CHIKV but could also neutralize it upon binding to its functional epitopes *in vivo.*

In the case of CHIKV, the level of neutralizing antibodies correlated with a protective immune response, which provides protection during challenge in the animals (Akahata et al., 2010; Weaver et al., 2012). In our study VLPs were shown to elicit a high titer of neutralizing antibodies that led to protection against CHIKV in neonatal mice. Therefore, this is in agreement with previous studies where CHIK- VLPs have been shown to elicit neutralizing antibodies (Akahata et al., 2010; Metz et al., 2013).

Cell-mediated immune response against different formulations of CHIK-VLPs was also evaluated in this study. The provision of an effective means to stimulate both the humoral and cell-mediated arms of the immune response is crucial for vaccine development. Hence, the present study demonstrates induction of efficient cell-mediated immune response by CHIK-VLPs is an important finding. Results of the cell-mediated response against CHIK-VLPs demonstrated the balanced Th1 and Th2 response. IL-2, TNF-α and IFN-γ mediate Th1 response and IL-4 and IL-10 mediate Th2 response. Higher expression of TNF-α, IL-10 and moderate expression of IL-2, IL-4 and IFN-γ indicated a balanced Th1/Th2 response. Significant up-regulation of TNF-α, IL-2 and elevated levels of IgG2a favored the Th1 response responsible to act against most of the pathogens, while the Th2 response involved the production of IL-4, IL-10 and enhanced the production of IgG1. The role of the cell-mediated immune response in protection against CHIKV has been studied earlier in wild-type mice (Gardner et al., 2010), where an elevated level of TNF-α and IFN-γ helps in protection against natural CHIKV infection (Schneider et al., 2008). The induction of a higher level of TNF-α and IFN-γ has been observed in mice immunized with different doses of CHIK-VLPs supporting the efficient generation of acell -mediate dimmune response similar to that of native CHIKV response.

In conclusion, our results showed that *P. pastoris*-expressed CHIK-VLPs are immunogenic and efficient at inducing virus-neutralizing antibodies and specific cellular responses in immunized mice. Considering the safety, reliability and also economic potential of the *Pichia* expression platform, our results indicate the feasibility of this system for large-scale and rapid production of safe and effective Chikungunya VLPs, which can serve as a vaccine candidate.

CHAPTER 8

SUMMARY OF CHIKUNGUNYA VIRUS-LIKE PARTICLES

Chikungunya is one of the most important re-emerging human arboviral infections of global significance. It is an acute mosquito-borne febrile arthritis caused by the Chikungunya virus (CHIKV), a member of *Alphavirus* belonging to the family *Togaviridae*. CHIKV is an enveloped, positive-strand RNA virus of approximately 12000 nucleotides. The genome of CHIKV is organized as: 5' cap-nsP1-nsP2-nsP3-nsP4-(junction region)- C-E3-E2-6K-E1-poly(A) 3'. The virus was isolated in 1952 from Tanzanian. The disease is characterized by abrupt onset of high fever, arthralgia, myalgia, headache, and rash. The typical clinical sign of the disease is poly-arthralgia which is very painful. The arthralgia may persist in a small proportion of cases for several months. In some patients, minor hemorrhagic signs such as epistaxis or gingivorrhagia have also been described.

CHIKV has re-emerged as an important pathogen causing epidemics in several parts of the world. Geographically, CHIKV is distributed in Africa, India, and South-East Asia. The virus appears to have spread from Africa to other parts of the world and caused epidemics in the Asian tropics. In Asia, CHIKV is transmitted from human to human mainly by *Ae. aegypti* and, to a lesser extent, by *Ae. albopictus* through an urban transmission cycle. In India, *Ae. aegypti* is the main vector, whereas the *Ae. albopictus* is considered as the main vector in Reunion and other islands of the Indian Ocean. Since the 1952 Tanzania outbreak, CHIKV has caused numerous outbreaks in East Africa (Tanzania and Uganda), in Austral Africa (Zimbabwe and South Africa), in West Africa (Senegal and Nigeria), and in Central Africa (Central African Republic and the Democratic Republic of the Congo). CHIKV emerged in the islands of the south-western Indian Ocean at the end of 2004. Later in 2005, the virus circulated in the other islands, i.e, Mayotte, Seychelles, Re´union and Mauritius. In India, the first outbreak of CHIK was recorded in 1963 in Kolkata, followed by sporadic epidemics in eastern coastal areas, namely Chennai, Pondicherry and Vellore in 1964, Visakhapatnam, Rajamundry and Kakinada in 1965, Nagpur in 1965 and Barsi in 1973. After a gap of almost 32 years, several states in India experienced massive outbreaks of CHIK during 2005–2006 affecting almost 1.39 million persons. The outbreaks continued for the next two consecutive years (2007 and 2008) affecting predominantly Kerala and Karnataka states, respectively.

The vector control measures that can play important role in the control of infection proved unsuccessful in many parts of the world. Currently, there are no licensed antivirals or vaccines available commercially. There is also a scarcity of reliable diagnostic kits in endemic areas, making disease management and virus transmission control extremely difficult. The routine laboratory diagnosis of CHKV infection is based on virus isolation, molecular assays (RT-PCR) and serology. Both virus isolation and RT-PCR though highly specific, are technically demanding and currently restricted to referral laboratories. Serologically, CHIKV diagnosis relies on the detection of IgM and IgG antibodies through ELISA and immunochromatography test (ICT). In view of large-scale epidemic potential of CHIKV, there is a need to develop fast high throughput serological diagnostic assays which are amenable to remote settings. The success of serological assays inherently depends on the quality of the antigen. Replacement of cell culture derived native CHIKV antigen by recombinant virus protein leads to improved specificity, however, the limitation includes compromised sensitivity, due to the availability of limited immunogenic epitopes.

Virus-Like particles (VLPs) are non-infectious, nanosized caged structures composed of viral structural proteins. The presence of complete structural proteins makes it an excellent antigen that strongly mimics the native virus. Currently, available commercial ELISA and ICT kits suffer from the issues of poor sensitivity and specificity and many products were withdrawn from the market (Prat et al., 2014). The VLPs-based diagnostic assay provides a promising alternative for the detection of CHIKV infection with a high degree of sensitivity and specificity.

Vaccination is the most effective way of protecting humans and limiting further CHIKV transmission. CHIKV infection is believed to induce life-long immunity through a protective antibody response (Tiwari et al., 2009), indicating that naive individuals could be protected for life, if a safe and efficacious vaccine induces a similar antibody response. Currently, there are no specific treatments (antiviral) or commercial vaccines for CHIKV infections available. However, the emergence of CHIKV and the clinical manifestation of the disease in humans have triggered vaccine development. The first vaccine prototype was a formalin-inactivated virus, developed by the United States Army Medical Research Institute of Infectious Diseases (USAMRIID). Although efficacious, a major drawback is that production of the virus must take place in costly, biosafety level 3 facilities. As an alternative, live-attenuated virus vaccines have been developed (Levitt et al., 1986). Live-attenuated virus vaccines have the advantage of inducing an efficient, balanced immune response, but have the drawback of the risk of reversion to virulence (Noad and Roy, 2003).

The prospect of live (attenuated) alphavirus vaccine development remains questionable due to vaccine-induced clinical manifestations and the undeniable risk of transmission by mosquito vectors, but most of all, the possible reversion to virulence. In addition to the 181/clone25 vaccine, a broad range of vaccine strategies have been described, including other live-attenuated virus vaccines (Partidos et al., 2012), chimeric virus vaccines (Wang et al., 2008), DNA vaccines (Mallilankaraman et al., 2011), adenoviral vectored vaccines (Wang et al., 2011), subunit protein vaccines (Kumar et al., 2012) and virus-like particle (VLP) formulations (Akahata et al., 2010). However, these vaccination strategies have their own specific complications in manufacturing, immunogenicity, safety, recombination and large-scale production (Kutzler et al., 2008). Recent studies have shown promising results in the development of a CHIK-VLPs-based vaccine. VLPs elicited a neutralizing antibody response against homologous and heterologous strains and protection against a high-dose CHIKV challenge (Akahata et al., 2010).

The continuous expansion of CHIKV and increase in human morbidity make it one of the most important emerging arboviruses. There is a demand to develop a safe and economical diagnostic assay for screening of a large number of patients during the time of epidemics. Further, a safe and effective CHIKV vaccine is clearly needed to protect humans and also to stop CHIKV transmission. Several strategies have been designed to combat CHIKV infections but none of these have been licensed yet and are not easily amenable to scale up. The purpose of this study is to design and develop a novel CHIKV immunogen that can be employed for both diagnostic and prophylactic applications.

Quality of antigen plays the most crucial role in the development of a diagnostic system. VLPs owing to their close conformational resemblance to the native virus provide the best quality of antigen further obviating biosafety concerns. It has also shown the ability to induce both humoral and cell-mediated immune responses. The Yeast (*Pichia pastoris*) based expression system is now widely adopted for the expression of viral proteins intended for both diagnostic and prophylactic applications.

Keeping in view these facts, the present study was undertaken to develop advanced VLPs- based new generation diagnostic and vaccine candidates with the following points:

A two-step purification strategy for Chikungunya virion using sucrose buoyant density gradient separation.

Heterologous expression and characterization of CHIK-VLPs using *Pichia pastoris*.

Evaluation of CHIK-VLPs as a diagnostic intermediate in serological diagnosis.

Evaluation of the immunogenic potential of CHIK-VLPs in BALB/c mice.

A Two-step Purification Strategy for Chikungunya Virion using Sucrose Buoyant Density Gradient Separation

Chikungunya virus has emerged as one of the most important and widespread arboviral infections of public health significance. Its recent emergence in both the old and new worlds generated immense interest among global researchers to develop suitable diagnostic and medical control measures. The virus purification is one of the most challenging areas for the development of any downstream research as either diagnostics or prophylaxis. An improved method for purifying the Chikungunya virus from the cell culture supernatant of infected African Green Monkey Kidney (Vero) cells is described.

It employs a combination of polyethylene glycol (PEG 6000) precipitation with sucrose gradient ultracentrifugation. The infected cell culture supernatant was precipitated using polyethylene glycol and concentrated virus was banded at the interface of 20-60% (w/v) discontinuous sucrose gradient using rate zonal ultracentrifugation. Using a combination of SDS-PAGE and western blotting techniques, CHIKV structural proteins were detected only in the fractions collected from the interface.

The authenticity of the purified Chikungunya virions was further confirmed by reverse transcriptase polymerase chain reaction (RT-PCR) and transmission electron microscopic (TEM) study. The developed method has immense application and is useful in making a large quantity of purified CHIKV for its characterization, virus morphological study and purification of CHIK- VLPs expressed from the heterologous system. This technique has been successfully utilized to standardize and purify native CHIKV antigen-based IgM ELISA that was used as a reference assay for comparative evaluation of other antigen-based ELISA in this study.

Heterologous Expression and Characterization of CHIK-VLPs using Pichia Pastoris

Virus-like particles (VLPs) are multistructured proteins that mimic the organization and conformation of native viruses but lack the viral genome. Therefore, they are noninfectious and potentially safer vaccine candidates and diagnostic antigens. Previously CHIK-VLPs have been expressed in mammalian and baculovirus insect cell expression systems and found to be effective as a vaccine candidate.

But these VLPs have some disadvantages; CHIK-VLPs based on a mammalian cell expression system are related to higher production cost and lower controllability and productivities. Moreover, in the baculovirus insect cell expression system, co-production of enveloped baculovirus particles contaminates the vaccine candidate and may impair the vaccine quality.

Moreover, baculovirus particles and VLPs are difficult to separate; VLPs produced in this system have to undergo either chemical inactivation treatments or several downstream processing steps to eliminate baculovirus infectivity that will subsequently increase the production cost. *Pichia* cells readily grow in suspension cultures, which is a benefit of the yeast expression system.

The *Pichia pastoris* (*P. pastoris*) yeast expression system used in this study offers several advantages for VLPs development: the techniques needed for molecular manipulation are simple, the ability to produce large-scale foreign proteins in their native conformation, operating costs are cheaper, simple chemical media and free from virus contamination, makes it an attractive alternative platform.

Recent studies demonstrated that CHIK-VLPs have antigenic specificity which was similar to native CHIKV. We employed the novel *Pichia* expression system to produce CHIK-VLPs. In this study, the gene encoding the complete structural polyprotein (C-E3- E2-6K-E1) was amplified in two overlapping fragments and fused at the natural restriction site. Further, the GS115 strain of *Pichia pastoris* was transformed with a yeast transfer vector having the C-E3-E2-6k-E1 gene. The multicopy integrants were processed for the expression of CHIK-VLPs. Expression parameters were optimized i.e. concentration of methanol was found to be 2 % and the time of VLPs harvest was 48 hrs.

We detected 50 kDa protein corresponding to E1 and/or E2 in the supernatant. Transmission electron microscopy revealed spherical particles with a 50- to 60-nm diameter in the supernatant that resembled the native CHIKV virions. The yield of purified VLPs was 60 ng/μl. These VLPs were found to react with serum raised against CHIKV-E2 protein, indicating that their antigenicity is similar to that of native CHIKV. These results indicated that CHIKV VLPs are morphologically and antigenically similar to the native CHIKV, suggesting that they have the potential for use in both chikungunya diagnosis and vaccine formulation.

Evaluation of CHIK-VLPs as a Diagnostic Intermediate in Serological Diagnosis

An indirect microplate IgM ELISA was standardized using the purified CHIK- VLPs, as antigen. The antigenicity of CHIK-VLPs was initially confirmed using rabbit polyclonal antibody raised against purified native CHIKV and recombinant E2 protein. This indicated its potential utility for the detection of anti-CHIKV IgM in patient sera. An indirect IgM ELISA protocol was optimized using 300 ng of CHIK-VLPs with minimal background. The comparative evaluation of CHIK-VLPs and rCHIK-E2 based ELISA revealed significantly higher mean O.D. values in CHIK-

VLPs based ELISA indicating its superiority over rCHIK-E2 antigen.

CHIK-VLPs were found to be most effective in terms of recognizing the CHIKV-specific IgM from patient's sera with 97% concordance, 97.29% sensitivity and 96.82% specificity compared to the standard purified CHIKV. No cross-reactivity was observed in the case of dengue and JE patient sera and also with healthy human sera. The most important advantage of this assay is that it can differentiate chikungunya infection from dengue fever, making it an extremely useful screening assay in many endemic areas where both dengue and chikungunya are co-circulating.

In conclusion, CHIK-VLPs-based IgM- ELISA described in this study was specific for the detection of anti-CHIKV IgM antibodies in human patient sera. Overall comparable sensitivity and specificity of the CHIK-VLPs-based IgM-ELISA achieved in this study offer a promising economical tool for clinical diagnosis as well as rapid surveillance of CHIKV infection.

Evaluation of the Immunogenic Potential of CHIK-VLPs in BALB/c Mice

Chikungunya virus (CHIKV) is a global health concern, due to its recent spread in both old and new worlds. So far, no CHIKV-specific licensed vaccine or drug is available. In this study, we report the production of Chikungunya Virus-Like particles (CHIK-VLPs) using a novel yeast expression system (*Pichia pastoris*) and its evaluation as a vaccine candidate.

The *in vitro* and *in vivo* evaluation of CHIK-VLPs as a prophylactic intermediate was determined in Balb/c mice. Induction of both humoral and cell-mediated immune responses was observed with different doses of CHIK-VLPs.

The humoral immune response was studied through different techniques like enzyme linked immunosorbent assay, IgG Isotyping and plaque reduction neutralization test. CHIK- VLPs were found to elicit a high titer of antibodies that are able to recognize native CHIKV. A higher level of IgG2a and IgG1 subtypes were identified as suggestive of balanced Th1/Th2 response.

Both *in vitro* and *in vivo* neutralization activity of CHIK-VLPs antibodies was observed even with low concentration, which shows its high specificity and neutralizing activity against CHIKV. Neonatal mice receiving anti-CHIK-VLPs antibodies were protected from the CHIKV challenge. Induction of cell-mediated immune response was confirmed through a higher level of TNF-α and IL-10 with a substantial level of IL- 2, IL-4 and IFN-γ indicating a balanced response.

This is the first report, where (CHIK- VLPs) have been expressed by *Pichia pastoris* and evaluated for their neutralizing activity against CHIKV. These promising results indicate the utility of CHIK-VLPs as a potential vaccine candidate against emerging CHIKV.

Conclusions

Chikungunya virions were successfully purified by an improved method using two steps with minimum impurities. The concentration and buoyant density gradient method followed in the present study particularly suits the purification of Chikungunya virus, which produce low virus titers. It may also find applications in purifying Chikungunya VLPs and viruses for its morphological characterization and evaluation of antigenicity.

The full structural polyprotein of CHIKV was successfully transformed into *P. pastoris* and the integrity of transgene were further confirmed by genomic DNA PCR. Clones that were resistant to higher concentrations of Geneticin also showed intensive bands in genomic DNA PCR and these results were in agreement with that of the Geneticin sensitivity assay.

The expression of CHIK-VLPs appeared to be better in the case of YPM. The optimum methanol concentration for better expression of CHIK-VLPs was found to be 2 %. The expressed protein yield was shown to increase up to 48 hrs after which the point protein concentration was stable showing that 48 hr post induction was the optimum time to harvest.

The structural polyprotein of CHIKV was fused with α- factor secretion signal of *Saccharomyces cerevisiae* under the control of methanol inducible *Pichia pastoris* alcohol oxidase 1 (AOX1) promoter in the pPIC9K yeast transfer vector. This α- factor secretion signal helps in secreted expression. Hence, CHIK-VLPs were secreted in the culture medium.

CHIK-VLPs were purified using discontinuous sucrose density gradient ultracentrifugation. SDS-PAGE analyses of different fractions revealed that the majority of CHIK-VLPs were localized at the 20-60% sucrose interface. The authenticity of CHIK-VLPs was examined *via* western blotting using different anti-CHIKV antibodies.

The average diameter of Chikungunya cores was found approximately 40 nm which is consistent with the reported size of the chikungunya virus and other alphaviruses. Thus, yeast-derived CHIK-VLPs are morphologically identical to CHIKV.

The overall comparable sensitivity and specificity of CHIK-VLPs-based IgM- ELISA achieved 97% in this study offers a promising economical tool for clinical diagnosis of CHIKV infection.

The potential of CHIK-VLPs to discriminate clinically similar Dengue samples make it a useful screening assay in endemic areas where Chikungunya and Dengue are co-circulating.

Both sensitivity and specificity of CHIK-VLPs-based ELISA were found to be higher compared to rCHIK-E2-based ELISA, indicating the superiority of VLPs as an antigen.

Yeast-derived CHIK-VLPs elicited both humoral and cell-mediated immune responses in mice. These VLPs generated a high titer of neutralizing antibodies that recognized native CHIKV. A dose-dependent antibody titer has been seen after booster doses. Immunization of different doses of CHIK-VLPs with FCA showed the balanced immune response with the approximately high and same amount of IgG1 and IgG2a.

The antibodies raised against CHIK-VLPs were highly specific and recognize native CHIKV and mainly bind to CHIKV antigen on neutralization. Immunized mice showed full protection and survival after the CHIKV challenge.

CHIK-VLPs induced an efficient cell-mediated immune response as observed by balanced Th1 and Th2 responses. Higher expression of TNF-α, IL-10 and moderate expression of IL-2, IL-4 and IFN-γ indicated a balanced Th1/Th2 response. A balanced Th1/Th2 response along with neutralizing antibody was observed, indicating the utility of CHIK-VLPs as a potential vaccine candidate.

The protective efficacy of CHIKV-VLPs against CHIKV was also evaluated. Neonatal mice that received anti-CHIK-VLPs antibodies were protected from CHIKV challenge as evident through reduced CHIKV-associated disease.

In conclusion, the present study was aimed at developing a cheaper and more economic platform to develop CHIK-VLPs. The potential of *P. pastoris* to express CHIK-VLPs has been shown for the first time. These CHIK-VLPs are morphologically similar to the native virion. An IgM ELISA-based diagnostic method for the detection of Chikungunya virus infection has been developed and evaluated. This assay has good sensitivity and specificity which suggests that the test can be used as an accurate tool for surveillance and early diagnosis of CHIKV infection in endemic areas. We also demonstrated that CHIK-VLPs are immunogenic and efficient in inducing virus-neutralizing antibodies and balancing Th1/Th2 response in immunized mice. Purified IgG from CHIK-VLPs immunized mice sera showed protection against CHIKV viremia and hind limb paralysis. Therefore, these results based on *in vitro* and *in-vivo* studies confirm the protective efficacy of CHIK-VLPs against the emerging Chikungunya virus and its potential as a future vaccine candidate.

REFERENCES

1. **Agarwal A**, **Singh AK, Sharma S,** et al. Application of Real-time RT-PCR in vector surveillance and assessment of replication kinetics of an emerging Novel ECSA genotype of Chikungunya virus in Aedes aegypti. J Virol Methods. 2013;193:419-425.
2. **Ahola T, Courderc T, Ng LF**, et al.Therapeutics and Vaccines Against Chikungunya Virus. Vector Borne Zoonotic Dis. 2015;15:250-257.
3. **Akahata W, Yang ZY, Andersen H**, et al. A virus-like particle vaccine for epidemic chikungunya virus protects nonhuman primates against infection. Nat Med. 2010;16:334- 8.
4. **Alessandra LP, Lai A, Cella E,** et al. Chikungunya virus, epidemiology, clinics and phylogenesis: A review. Asian Pac J Trop Med. 2014;12:925-932.
5. **Andersson, H, Barth BU, Ekström M,** et al. Oligomerization-dependent folding of the membrane fusion protein of Semliki Forest virus. J Virol. 1997;71:9654-63.
6. **Arankalle VA, Shrivastava S, Cherian S**, et al. Genetic divergence of Chikungunya viruses in India (1963-2006) with special reference to the 2005-2006 explosive epidemic. J Gen Virol. 2007; 88:1967–1976.

7. **Athmaram TN, Saraswat S, Misra P,** et al. A two-step purification strategy for Chikungunya virions purification using sucrose buoyant density gradient separation. J Virol Research. 2013;2:18-21.

8. **Barrett ADT**. Arboviruses: alphaviruses, flaviviruses and bunyaviruses. In: Greenwood D, Slack RCB, Peutherer JF (editors). Medical microbiology. London: Churchill Livingstone; 2002;16:484-501.

9. **Bazan SB, de Alencar Muniz Chaves A, Aires KA**, et al. Expression and characterization of HPV-16 L1 capsid protein in *Pichia pastoris*. Arch. Virol. 2009;154:1609–1617.

10. **Bobrowicz P**, **Davidson RC, Li H,** et al. Engineering of an artificial glycosylation pathway blocked in core oligosaccharide assembly in the yeast *Pichia pastoris*: production of complex humanized glycoproteins with terminal galactose. Glycobiology. 2004;14:757–766.

11. **Borgherini G, Patrice Poubeau1, Annie Jossaume,** et al. Persistent arthralgia associated with Chikungunya virus: a study of 88 adult patients on reunion island. Clinical infectious diseases: an official publication of the Infectious Diseases Society of America. 2008;47:469–475.

12. **Brooks GF**, Human arboviral infections. In: Jawetz. Melnick and Adelberg's Medical microbiology. Singapore: Mc Graw Hill, 2004; 23:514-524.

13. **Burke DS, Nisalak A, Nimmannitya S,** et al. Disappearance of Chikungunya virus from Bangkok. Trans R Soc Trop Med Hyg. 1985;79:419–420.

14. **Byrne B**. *Pichia pastoris* as an expression host for membrane protein structural biology. Curr Opin Struct Biol. 2015;32:9-17.

15. **Caglioti C, Lalle E, Castilletti C, et al.** Chikungunya virus infection: an overview. New Microbiol. 2013;36:211-27.

16. **Carey DE**. Chikungunya and dengue: A case of mistaken identity? J Hist Med Allied Sci. 1971;26:243–262.

17. **Carletti F, Chiappini R, Ippolito G,** et al. Rapid detection and quantification of Chikungunya virus by a one-step reverse transcription polymerase chain reaction real- time assay. Am J Trop Med Hyg. 2007;77:521-524.

18. Casadaban M, Martinez-Arias A, Shapira SK, et al. Beta-galactosidase gene fusions for analyzing gene expression in *Escherichia coli* and yeast. J.,Methods Enzymol. 1983;100:293–308.

19. Cecilia D. Current status of Dengue and Chikungunya in India. WHO South-East Asia J Public Health 2014;3:22–27.

20. Cekinovic D, Golemac M, Pugel EP, et al. Passive immunization reduces murine cytomegalovirus-induced brain pathology in newborn mice. J Virol. 2008;82:12172-80.

21. Cereghino JL and Cregg JM. Heterologous protein expression in the methylotrophic yeast *Pichia pastoris*. FEMS Microbiology Reviews. 2000;24:45-66.

22. Chang LJ, Dowd KA2, Mendoza FH, et al. Safety and tolerability of chikungunya virus-like particle vaccine in healthy adults: a phase 1 dose-escalation trial. Lancet 2014;384:2046-52.

23. Chastel C. Human infections in Cambodia by the chikungunya virus or an apparently closely related agent. I. Clinical aspects. Isolations and identification of the viruses. Serology. Bull Soc Pathol Exot Filiales. 1963;56:892–915.

24. Cho B, Kim J, Cho JE, et al. Expression of the Capsid protein of chikungunya virus in a baculovirus for serodiagnosis of chikungunya disease. J Virol methods. 2008a;154:154- 159.

25. Cho B, Jeon BY, Kim J, et al. Expression and Evalution of chikungunya Virus E1 and E2 Envelope proteins for serodiagnosis of Chikungunya virus infection. Yonsei Med J. 2008b;49:828-835.

26. Choi BK, Bobrowicz P, Davidson RC, et al. Use of combinatorial genetic libraries to humanize N-linked glycosylation in the yeast *Pichia pastoris*. Appl Biol Sci 2003;100:5022–5027.

27. Chow A, Her Z, Ong EK, et al. Persistent arthralgia induced by chikungunya virus infection is associated with interleukin-6 and granulocyte macrophage colony-stimulating factor. J Infect Dis. 2011;203:149-57.

28. Chevillon C, Briant L, Renaud F, et al. Review, The Chikungunya threat, an ecological and evolutionary perspective. Cell. 2007;12:80-88.

29. Cregg JM, Madden KR. Development of transformation systems and construction of methanol-utilisation-defective mutants of *Pichia* *pastoris* by gene disruption. In Biological Research on Industrial Yeast. 1987;2:1-18.

30. **Cregg JM, Vedvick TS, Raschke WC**. Recent advances in the expression of foreign genes in *Pichia pastoris*. Biotechnology 1993;11:905-910.
31. **Cregg JM**, **Cereghino JL, Shi J, Higgins DR,** et al. Recombinant protein expression in *Pichia pastoris*. Mol Biotechnol. 2000;16:23-52.
32. **Couderc T, Chrétien F, Schilte C,** et al. A mouse model for Chikungunya: young age and inefficient type-I interferon signaling are risk factors for severe disease. PLoS Pathog. 2008;4:e29.
33. **Cui F, Raymond M, Qiao CL,** et al. Insecticide resistance in vector mosquitoes in China. Pest Manag Sci. 2006;62:1013-1022.
34. **Dash PK, Parida MM, Santhosh SR**, et al. East Central South African genotype as the causative agent in reemergence of chikungunya outbreak in India. Vector Borne Zoonotic Dis. 2007;7:519–27.
35. **Dash PK, Parida MM, Saxena P,** et al. Reemergence of dengue virus type-3 (subtype- III) in India: Implications for increased incidences of DHF and DSS. Virol J. 2006;3:55. **Dash PK, Tiwari M, Santhosh SR, et al.** RNA interference mediated inhibition of Chikungunya virus replication in mammalian cells. Biochem Biophys Res Commun. 2008;376:718–722.
36. **Diallo M, Thonnon J, Traore-Lamizana M, Fontenille D**, et al. Vectors of Chikungunya virus in Senegal: current data and transmission cycles. Am J Trop Med Hyg. 1999;60:281–286.
37. **Ding MX, Schlesinger MJ.** Evidence that Sindbis virus NSP2 is an autoprotease which processes the virus nonstructural polyprotein. Virology. 1989;171:280-4.
38. **Dupont-Rouzeyrol M, Caro V, Guillaumot L**, et al. Chikungunya virus and the mosquito vector *Aedes aegypti* in New Caledonia (South Pacific Region). Vector Borne Zoonotic Dis 2012;12:1036–1041.
39. **Dupis-Maguiragal, Noret M, Brun S,** et al. Chikungunya disease: infection-associated markers from the acute to the chronic phase of arbovirus-induced arthralgia. PLoS Negl. Trop. Dis. 2012;6:e1446.
40. **Edwards, CJ, Welch SR, Chamberlain J,** et al. Molecular diagnosis and analysis of Chikungunya virus. J Clin Virol. 2007;39:271-5.

41. **Edelman R, Tacket CO, Wasserman SS,** et al. Phase II safety and immunogenicity study of live chikungunya virus vaccine TSIGSD-218. Am J Trop Med Hyg 2000;62:681-5.

42. **Eckels KH, Harrison VR, Hetrick FM.** Chikungunya virus vaccine prepared by Tween- ether extraction. Appl Microbiol. 1970;19:321-5.

43. **Faragher SG, Meek AD, Rice CM,** et al. Genome sequences of a mouse-avirulent and a mouse-virulent strain of Ross River virus. Virology. 1988;163:509-26.

44. **Foo DG, Alonso S, Chow VT,** et al. Passive protection against lethal enterovirus 71 infection in newborn mice by neutralizing antibodies elicited by a synthetic peptide. Microbes Infect. 2007;11:1299-306.

45. **Gasque P, Couderc T, Lecuit M,** et al. Chikungunya virus pathogenesis and immunity. Vector Borne Zoonotic Dis. 2015;15:241–249.

46. **Gardner J, Anraku I, Le TT,** et al. Chikungunya virus arthritis in adult wild-type mice. J Virol. 2010;84:8021-32.

47. **Garoff, H, Sjöberg M, Cheng RH.** Budding of alphaviruses. Virus Res. 2004;106:103- 16.

48. **Garmashova N, Gorchakov R, Volkova E,** et al. The Old World and New World alphaviruses use different virus specific proteins for induction for transcriptional shutoff. J.Virol. 2007;81:2472-2484.

49. **Gerngross TU**. Advances in the production of human therapeutic proteins in yeasts and filamentous fungi. Nature Biotechnol. 2004;22:1409-1414.

50. **Gibbons, DL, Ahn A, Chatterjee PK,** et al. Formation and characterization of the trimeric form of the fusion protein of Semliki forest virus. J Virol. 2000;74:7772-80.

51. **Grgacic EV, Anderson DA.** Virus-like particles: passport to immune recognition. Methods. 2006;40:60-5.

52. **Griffin D, Levine B, Tyor W,** et al. The role of antibody in recovery from alphavirus encephalitis. Immunol Rev. 1997;159:155-61.

53. **Griffin D,** et al. Alphaviruses In: Fields BN, Knipe DM, PM H, editors. Field Virology. Philadelphia: Lippincott-Williams & Wilkins. 2007;5:1023–1068.

54. **Grivard P, Le Roux K, Laurent P,** et al. Molecular and serological diagnosis of Chikungunya virus infection. Pathol. Biol. 2007;55:490–494.

55. **Gorchakov R, Wang E, Leal G,** et al. Attenuation of chikungunya virus vaccine strain 181/clone 25 is determined by two amino acid substitutions in the E2 envelope glycoprotein. J Virol. 2012;86:6084-96.
56. **Guarna MM, Lesnicki GJ, Tam BM,** et al. On-line monitoring and control of methanol concentration in shake-flask cultures of *Pichia pastoris*. Biotechnol Bioeng. 1997;56:279– 286.
57. **Gubler DJ, Reiter P, Ebi KL,** et al. Climate variability and change in the United States: potential impacts on vector- and rodent-borne diseases. Environ Health Perspect. 2001;2:223-233.
58. **Harrison VR, Eckels KH, Bartelloni PJ,** et al. Production and evaluation of a formalin- killed chikungunya vaccine. J Immunol. 1971;107:643-7.
59. **Hasebe F, Parquet MC, Pandey BD**, et al. Combined detection and genotyping of Chikungunya virus by a specific reverse transcription-polymerase chain reaction. J Med Virol. 2002;67:370–374.
60. **Her Z, Malleret B, Chan M,** et al. Active infection of human blood monocytes by Chikungunya Virus Triggers an Innate Immune response. J. Immunol. 2010;184:5903-13. **Hervas-Stubbs S, Rueda P, Lopez L,** et al. Insect baculoviruses strongly potentiate adaptive immune responses by inducing type I IFN. J Immunol. 2007;178:2361-9.
61. **Hitzeman RA, Hagie FE, Levine HL,** et al. Expression of a human gene for interferon in yeast. Nature. 1981;293:717–732.
62. **Hitzeman RA, Chen CY, Dowbenko DJ,** et al. Use of heterologous and homologous signal sequences for secretion of heterologous proteins from yeast. Methods Enzymol. 1990;185:421–440.
63. **Hoke CH Jr, Pace-Templeton J, Pittman P,** et al. US Military contributions to the global response to pandemic chikungunya. Vaccine. 2012;30:6713–6720.
64. **Horwood PF, Reimer LJ, Dagina R,** et al. Outbreak of chikungunya virus infection, Vanimo, Papua New Guinea. Emerg Infect Dis. 2013b;19:1535–1538.
65. **Hunt AR, Frederickson S, Maruyama T,** et al. The first human epitope map of the alphaviral E1 and E2 proteins reveals a new E2 epitope with significant virus neutralizing activity. PLoS Negl Trop Dis. 2010;4:e739.

66. **Jadhav M, Namboodripad M, Carman RH,** et al. Chikungunya disease in infants and children in Vellore: a report of clinical and haematological features of virologically proved cases. Indian J Med Res.1965;53:764–776.

67. **Jahic M, Gustavsson M, Jansen AK,** et al. Analysis and control of proteolysis of a fusion protein in *Pichia pastoris* fed-batch processes. Bio Technology. 2003;102:42–53.

68. **Jahrling PB, Hesse RA, Anderson,** et al. Opsonization of alphaviruses in hamsters. J Med Virol. 1983;12:1-16.

69. **Jeandel P, Josse R, Durand JP.** Exotic viral arthritis: role of alphavirus. Med Trop. 2004;64:81-88.

70. **Joseph AY, Babu VS, Dev SS,** et al. Rapid detection and characterization of chikungunya virus by RT-PCR in febrile patients from Kerala, India. Indian J Exp Biol. 2008;46:573–578.

71. **Jupp PG, McIntosh BM.** *Aedes furcifer* and other mosquitoes as vectors of chikungunya virus at Mica, northeastern Transvaal, South Africa. J Am Mosq Control Assoc. 1990;6:415-420.

72. **Kam YW, Ong EK, Rénia L, et al.** Immuno-biology of Chikungunya and implications for disease intervention. Microbes Infect. 2009;11:1186-96.

73. **Kam YW, Lee WW, Simarmata D,** et al. Longitudinal analysis of the human antibody response to chikungunya virus infection: implications for serodiagnosis and vaccine development. J Virol. 2012a ;86:13005-15.

74. **Kam YW, Lum FM, Teo TH,** et al. Early neutralizing IgG response to chikungunya virus in infected patients targets a dominant linear epitope on the E2 glycoprotein. EMBO Mol Med. 2012b;4:330-43.

75. **Kam YW, Simarmata D, Chow A,** et al. Early appearance of neutralizing immunoglobulin G3 antibodies is associated with chikungunya virus clearance and long- term clinical protection. J Infect Dis. 2012c;205:1147-54.

76. **Kashyap RS, Morey SH, Ramteke SS,** et al. Diagnosis of Chikungunya fever in an Indian Population by an Indirect Enzyme Linked Immunosorbent Assay. Clin Vaccine Immunol. 2010;5:291-297.

77. **Kaufman RJ**. Selection and coamplification of heterologous genes in mammalian cells.Methods Enzymol.1990;185:537–566.

78. **Kielian MC, Helenius A.** Role of cholesterol in fusion of semliki forest virus with membranes. J Virol. 1984;52:281-3.

79. **Khan AH, Morita K, Parquet Md Mdel C,** et al. Complete nucleotide sequence of Chikungunya virus and evidence for an internal polyadenylation site. Gen Virol, 2002;83:3075-3084.

80. **Khan M, Dhanwani R, Kumar JS,** et al. Comparative Evaluation of the Diagnostic Potential of Recombinant Envelope Proteins and Native Cell Culture Purified Viral Antigens of Chikungunya Virus. J. Med. Virol. 2014;86:1169–1175.

81. **Kit LS.** Emerging and re-emerging diseases in Malaysia. Asia Pac J Public Health. 2002;14:6–8.

82. **Konishi E, Hotta S**. Studies on structural proteins of Chikungunya Virus. I. Separation of three species of proteins and their preliminary characterization. Microbiol Immunol. 1980;24:419-28.

83. **Kornfeld R, Kornfeld S.** Assembly of asparagine-linked oligosaccharides. Annu. Rev. Biochem. 1985;54:631–664.

84. **Kuhn RJ**. *Togaviridae*: the viruses and their replication. Philadelphia, PA: Lippincott, Williams and Wilkins. 2007;7:1001–22.

85. **Kukuruzinska MA, Bergh ML, Jackson BJ.** Protein glycosylation in yeast. Annu. Rev. Biochem. 1987;56:915–944.

86. **Kumar J, Khan M, Gupta G,** et al. Production, characterization, and application of monoclonal antibodies specific to recombinant (E2) structural protein in antigen-capture ELISA for clinial diagnosis of Chikungunya virus. Viral immunol. 2012a;25:153-60.

87. **Kumar M, Sudeep AB, Arankalle VA.** Evaluation of recombinant E2 protein-based and whole-virus inactivated candidate vaccines against chikungunya virus. Vaccine. 2012b;30:6142-9.

88. **Kutzler MA, Weiner DB.** DNA vaccines: ready for prime time? Nat Rev Genet. 2008;10:776-88.

89. **Laemmli UK**. Cleavage of structural proteins during the assembly of the head of bacteriophage T4. Nature. 1970;227:680-5.

90. **Lam SK, Chua KB, Hooi PS,** et al. Chikungunya infection—an emerging disease in Malaysia. Southeast Asian J Trop Med Public Health. 2001;32:447-451.

91. **Laras K, Sukri NC, Larasati RP,** et al. Tracking the reemergence of epidemic chikungunya virus in Indonesia. Trans R Soc Trop Med Hyg. 2005;99:128-141.

92. **Laurent P, Le Roux K, Grivard P,** et al. Development of a sensitive real-time reverse transcriptase PCR assay with an internal control to detect and quantify chikungunya virus. Clin Chem. 2007;53:1408–1414.

93. **Leathers V, Tanguay R, Kobayashi M,** et al. A phylogenetically conserved sequence within viral 3' untranslated RNA pseudoknots regulates translation. Mol Cell Bio. 1993;13:5331-5347.

94. **Lemm JA, Rümenapf T, Strauss EG,** et al. Polypeptide requirements for assembly of functional sindbis virus replication complexes: a model for the temporal regulation of minus- and plus-strand RNA synthesis. Embo J. 1994;13:2925-34.

95. **Leparc-Goffart I, Nougairede A, Cassadou S,** et al. Chikungunya in the Americas. Lancet. 2014;383:514.

96. **Leroux-Roels G**. Old and new adjuvants for hepatitis B vaccines; Med Microbiol Immunol. 2015;204:69–78.

97. **Levitt NH, Ramsburg HH, Hasty SE,** et al. Development of an attenuated strain of chikungunya virus for use in vaccine production. Vaccine. 1986;4:157-62.

98. **Lewthwaite P, Vasanthapuram R, Osborne JC,** et al. Chikungunya Virus and Central Nervous System Infections in Children, India. Emerg Infec Dis . 2009;15:329-331.

99. **Litzba N, Schuffenecker I, Zeller H,** et al. Evaluation of the first commercial chikungunya virus indirect immunofluorescence test. J Virol Methods. 2008;149:175- 179.

100. **Lobigs M, Zhao HX, Garoff H.** Function of Semliki Forest virus E3 peptide in virus assembly: replacement of E3 with an artificial signal peptide abolishes spike heterodimerization and surface expression of E1. J Virol. 1990;64:4346-55.

101. **Lum FM, Ng LF**. Cellular and molecular mechanisms of chikungunya pathogenesis. Antiviral Research. 2015;120:165-74.

102. **Lundstrom K, Wagner R, Reinhart C, Desmyter A,** et al. Structural genomics on membrane proteins: comparison of more than 100 GPCRs in 3 expression systems. J Struct Funct Genomics. 2006;7:77-91.

103. **Macauley-Patrick S, Fazenda ML, McNeil B** et al. Heterologous protein production using the *Pichia pastoris* expression system. Yeast. 2005;22:249–270.

104. **Maina CV, Riggs PD, Grandea AG 3rd,** et al. An *Escherichia coli* vector to express and purify foreign proteins by fusion to and separation from maltose-binding protein. Gene. 1988;74:365–373.

105. **Makrides SC**. Strategies for achieving high-level expression of genes in *Escherichia coli*. Microbiol Rev. 1996;60:512-38

106. **Mallilankaraman K, Shedlock DJ, Bao H,** et al. A DNA vaccine against chikungunya virus is protective in mice and induces neutralizing antibodies in mice and nonhuman primates. PLoS Negl Trop Dis. 2011;5:e928.

107. **Mani S, Tripathi L, Raut R,** et al. *Pichia pastoris*-Expressed Dengue 2 Envelope Forms Virus-Like Particles without Pre-Membrane Protein and Induces High Titer Neutralizing Antibodies. PLoS ONE. 2013;8:e64595.

108. **Marchette NJ, Rudnick A, Garcia R,** et al. Alphaviruses in Peninsular Malaysia. I. Virus isolations and animal serology. Southeast Asian J Trop Med Public Health. 1978 ;9:317–329.

109. **Marston FA, Hartley DL.** Solubilization of protein aggregates. Methods Enzymol. 1990;182:264–276.

110. **McClain DJ, Pittman PR, Ramsburg HH,** et al. Immunologic interference from sequential administration of live attenuated alphavirus vaccines. J Infect Dis. 1998;177: 634–641.

111. **Metz SW, Geertsema C, Martina BE,** et al. Functional processing and secretion of chikungunya virus E1 and E2 glycoproteins in insect cells. Virol. J. 2011;8:353.

112. **Metz SW, Gardner J, Geertsema C,** et al. Effective chikungunya virus-like particle vaccine produced in insect cells. PLoS Negl Trop Dis. 2013;**7**:e2124.

113. **Mourya DT, Thakare JR, Gokhale MD,** et al. Isolation of chikungunya virus from *Aedes aegypti* mosquitoes collected in the town of Yawat, Pune District, Maharashtra State, India. Acta Virol. 2001;45:305–309.

114. **Muthumani K, Lankaraman KM, Laddy DJ,** et al. Immunogenicity of novel consensus-based DNA vaccines against chikungunya virus. Vaccine. 2008;26:5128-34.

115. **National Vector Borne Disease Control Programme**. Chikungunya fever. 2013; http://nvbdcp.gov.in/chikun-status.html - accessed 16 March 2014.

116. **Noad R, Roy P.** Virus-like particles as immunogens. Trends Microbiol. 2003;11:438-44. **Nimmannitya S, Halstead SB, Cohen SN,** et al. Dengue and chikungunya virus infection in man in Thailand, 1962–1964. I. Observations on hospitalized patients with hemorrhagic fever. Am J Trop Med Hyg. 1969;18:954–971.

117. **Nur YA, Groen J, Heuvelmans H,** et al. An outbreak of West Nile fever among migrants in Kisangani, Democratic Republic of Congo. Am J Trop Med Hyg. 1999;61:885–888.

118. **Ong RY, Lum FM, Lisa FP.** The fine line between protection and pathology in neurotropic flavivirus and alphavirus infections. Fut. Virol. 2014;9:313–330.

119. **O'Reilly**. Baculovirus Expression System – A Laboratory Manual, Oxford University Press, New York, 1992.

120. **Padbidri VS, Gnaneswar TT.** Epidemiological investigations of chikungunya epidemic at Barsi, Maharashtra state, India. J Hyg Epidemiol Microbiol Immunol. 1979;23:445– 451.

121. **Pan American Health Organization**. Number of reported cases of chikungunya fever in the Americas.2015.Available at http://www.paho.org/hq/index.php?option=com_topics&vi

122. ew=article&id=343&Itemid=40931

123. **Panning M, Charrel RN, Donoso Mantke O,** et al. Coordinated implementation of Chikungunya virus reverse transcription-PCR. Emerg Infect Dis. 2009;15:469–471.

124. **Palmer EL and Martin ML**. Electron Microscopy in Viral Diagnosis, CRC Press, Boca Raton, Florida. 1988.

125. **Parida MM, Santhosh SR, Dash PK,** et al. Rapid and real-time detection of chikungunya virus by reverse transcription loop-mediated isothermal amplification assay. J Clin Microbial. 2007;45:351–357.

126. **Parrott MM1, Sitarski SA, Arnold RJ,** et al. Role of conserved cysteines in the alphavirus E3 protein. J. Virol. 2009;83:2584 –2591..

127. **Partidos CD, Paykel J, Weger J,** et al. Cross-protective immunity against o'nyong- nyong virus afforded by a novel recombinant chikungunya vaccine. Vaccine. 2012;30:4638-43.

128. **Pastorino B, Muyembe-Tamfum JJ, Bessaud M,** et al. Epidemic resurgence of Chikungunya virus in democratic Republic of the Congo: Identification of a new central African strain. J Med Virol. 2004;74:277–282.

129. **Pastorino B1, Bessaud M, Grandadam M,** et al. Development of a TaqMan RT-PCR assay without RNA extraction step for the detection and quantification of African Chikungunya viruses. J Virol Methods. 2005;124:65-71.

130. **Pavri KM.** Presence of chikungunya antibodies in human sera collected from Calcutta and Jamshedpur before 1963. Indian J Med Res. 1964;52:698–702.

131. **Pedersen CE Jr, Eddy GA.** Separation, isolation, and immunological studies of the structural proteins of Venezuelan equine encephalomyelitis virus. J Virol. 1974;14:740-4. **Peyrefitte CN, Rousset D, Pastorino BA**, et al. Chikungunya virus, Cameroon, 2006. Emerg Infect Dis. 2007;13: 768–71.

132. **Peyrefitte CN, Bessaud M, Pastorino BA,** et al. Circulation of Chikungunya virus in Gabon, 2006–2007. J Med Virol. 2008;80:430–33.

133. **Pfeffer M, Linssen B, Parke MD,** et al. Specific detection of Chikungunya virus using a RT-PCR/nested PCR combination. J Vet Med B Infect Dis Vet Public Health. 2002;49:49–54.

134. **Plante K, Wang E, Partidos CD,** et al. Novel chikungunya vaccine candidate with an IRES-based attenuation and host range alteration mechanism. PLoS Pathog. 2011;7:e1002142.

135. **Powers AM, Brault AC, Shirako Y,** et al. Evolutionary relationships and systematics of the alphaviruses. J. Virol. 2001;75:10118–10131.

136. **Prat CM, Flusin O, Panella A,** et al. Evaluation of commercially available serologic diagnostic tests for Chikungunya virus. Emerg Infect Dis. 2014;12:2129-32

137. **Raemaekers RJ1, de Muro L, Gatehouse JA,** et al. Functional phytohemagglutinin (PHA) and *Galanthus nivalis* agglutinin (GNA) expressed in *Pichia pastoris*-correct N- terminal processing and secretion of heterologous proteins expressed using the PHA-E signal peptide. Eur J Biochem. 1999;265:394-403.

138. **Rai M, Padh H.** Expression systems for production of heterologous proteins. Current Science 2001 Current science, 2001;80: 225-238.

139. **Rao TR.** Recent epidemics caused by Chikungunya virus in India, 1963–1965. Sci Cult. 1966;32:215–220.

140. **Ravi V**. Re-emergence of chikungunya virus in India. Indian J Med Microbiol. 2006;24:83-84.

141. Reiter P, Fontenille D, Paupy C, et al. Aedes albopictus as an epidemic vector of chikungunya virus, another emerging problem? Lancet Infect Dis. 2006;6:463-464.

142. Rezza G, Nicoletti L, Angelini R, et al. CHIKV study group. Infection with Chikungunya virus in Italy: an outbreak in a temperate region. Lancet. 2007;370:1840- 1846.

143. Rianthavorn P, Wuttirattanakowit N, Prianantathavorn K, et al. Evaluation of a rapid assay for detection of IgM antibodies to chikungunya. Southeast Asian J. Trop. Med. Pub. Health. 2010;41:92–96.

144. Rodrigues FM, Patankar MR, Banerjee K, et al. Etiology of the 1965 epidemic of febrile illness in Nagpur city, Maharashtra State, India. Bull World Health Organ 1972;46:173–179.

145. Roehrig JT, Gorski D, Schlesinger MJ. Guidelines for Plaque-Reduction Neutralization Testing of Human Antibodies to Dengue Viruses. Viral Immunol. 2008;21:123–132.

146. Roldão A, Mellado MC, Castilho LR, et al. Virus-like particles in vaccine development. Expert Rev. Vaccines. 2010;9:1149–1176.

147. Romanos MA, Scorer CA, Clare JJ.. Foreign gene expression in yeast: a review. Yeast. 1992;8:423-488.

148. Romanos MA. Advances in the use of *Pichia pastoris* for high-level gene expression. Curr Opin Biotechnol. 1995;6:527-533.

149. Rueda P, Fominaya J, Langeveld JP, et al. Effect of different baculovirus inactivation procedures on the integrity and immunogenicity of porcine parvovirus-like particles. Vaccine. 2000;19;726-34.

150. Sambrook J, Fritsch EF, Maniatis T. Molecular Cloning: A Laboratory Manual. Cold Spring Harbor Laboratory Press, Nova York. 1989.

151. Sam IC, Kamarulzaman A, Ong GS, et al. Chikungunya virus-associated death in Malaysia. Trop Biomed. 2010;27:343–347.

152. Sam IC, Kümmerer BM, Chan YF, et al. Updates on Chikungunya Epidemiology, Clinical Disease, and Diagnostics. Vector Borne Zoonotic Dis. 2015;15:223-230.

153. Santhosh SR, Parida MM, Dash PK, et al. Development and evaluation of SYBR Green I-based one-step real-time RT-PCR assay for detection and quantification of Chikungunya virus. J. Clin. Virol. 2007;39:188-193.

154. **Sarkar JK, Chatterjee SN, Chakravarty SK,** et al. The Causative agent of Calcutta haemorrhagic fever: chikungunya or dengue. Bull Calcutta Sch Trop Med.1965;13:53-54. **Saxena S, Singh M, Mishra N,** et al. Resurgence of chikungunya virus in India: an emerging threat. Euro Surveill. 2006;11:E060810.2.

155. **Schneider BS, Higgs S.** The enhancement of arbovirus transmission and disease by mosquito saliva is associated with modulation of the host immune response. Trans. R. Soc. Trop. Med. Hyg. 2008;102:400–408.

156. **Schwarz B, Douglas T.** Development of virus-like particles for diagnostic and prophylactic biomedical applications. Wiley Interdiscip Rev Nanomed Nanobiotechnol 2015;7:722-35.

157. **Schwartz O**, **Albert ML.** Biology and pathogenesis of chikungunya virus. Nature Reviews Microbiology. 2010;8:491-500.

158. **Shah KV, Gibbs CJ, Banerjee G**. Virological investigation of the epidemic of haemorrhagic fever in Calcutta: isolation of three strains of Chikungunya virus. Indian J Med Res. 1964;52:676-83.

159. **Schuffenecker I**, **Iteman I, Michault A,** et al. Genome microevolution of Chikungunya Viruses causing the Indian Ocean outbreak. PLOS Med. 2006;3:e263.

160. **Scorer CA, Clare JJ, McCombie WR**, et al. Rapid selection using G418 of high cofly number transformants of *Pichia pastoris* for high-level foreign gene expression. Biotechnology. 1994;12:181-184.

161. **Shatzman AR and Rosenberg M**. Expression, identification, and characterization of recombinant gene products in *Escherichia coli*. Methods Enzymol. 1987;152:661–673.

162. **Shapiro AL, Viñuela E, Maizel JV Jr.** Molecular weight estimation of polypeptide chains by electrophoresis in SDS-polyacrylamide gels. Biochem Biophys Res Commun. 1967;28:815-20.

163. **Shukla J, Khan M, Tiwari M,** et al. Development and evaluation of antigen capture ELISA for early clinical diagnosis of Chikungunya. Diagn Micr Infec Dis. 2009;65:142– 149.

164. **Silberbach M, Maier B, Zimmermann M,** et al. Glucose oxidation by *Gluconobacter oxydans*: characterization in shaking flasks, scale-up and optimization of the pH profile. Appl Microbiol Biotechnol. 2003;62:92–98.

165. **Simizu B, Yamamoto K, Hashimoto K,** et al. Structural proteins of Chikungunya virus. J. Virol. 1984;51:254-258.

166. **Simon F, Savini H, Parola P.**. Chikungunya: a paradigm of emergence and globalization of vectorborne diseases. Med. Clin North Am. 2008;92:1323–1343.

167. **Sourisseau M, Schilte C, Casartelli N**, et al. Characterization of re-emerging chikungunya virus. PLoS Pathog. 2007;3:e89.

168. **Stephen Higgs and Vanlandingham Dana**. Chikungunya virus and Its mosquito vectors; Vector- born and Zoonotic Disease 2015;15:231-240.

169. **Strauss EG and Strauss JH.** Structure and replication of the alphavirus genome. In: S. Schlesinger and M.J. Schlesinger, Editors, The Togaviridae and Flaviridae , 1986;35–90 **Strauss JH and Strauss EG** Evolution of RNA viruses. Annual Review of Microbiology. 1988;42:657-683.

170. **Strauss EG and Strauss JH**. Identification of antigenically important domains in the glycoproteins of Sindbis virus by analysis of antibody escape variants. J Virol. 1991;65:4654-64.

171. **Strauss JH and Strauss EG.** The alphaviruses: gene expression, replication, and evolution. Microbiol Rev. 1994;58:491–562.

172. **Taubitz W, Cramer JP, Kapaun A,** et al. Chikungunya fever in travelers: clinical presentation and course. Clin Infect Dis. 2007;45:e1-4.

173. **Thaikruea L, Charearnsook O, Reanphumkarnkit S,** et al. Chikungunya in Thailand: a re-emerging disease? Southeast Asian J Trop Med Public Health. 1997;28:359–364.

174. **Thaung U, Ming CK, Swe T,** et al. Epidemiological features of dengue and chikungunya infections in Burma. Southeast Asian J Trop Med Public Health. 1975;6 :276–283.

175. **Thein S, La Linn M, Aaskov J,** et al. Development of a simple indirect enzyme-linked immunosorbent assay for the detection of immunoglobulin M antibody in serum from patients following an outbreak of chikungunya virus infection in Yangon, Myanmar. Trans R Soc Trop Med Hyg. 1992;86:438–442.

176. **Tiwari M, Parida M, Santhosh SR,** et al. Assessment of immunogenic potential of Vero adapted formalin inactivated vaccine derived from

novel ECSA genotype of chikungunya virus. Vaccine. 2009;27:2513-22.

177. **Vanlandingham DL, Hong C, Klingler K,** et al. Differential inactivities of o'nyong- nyong and Chikungunya virus isolates in *Anopheles gambiae* and *Aedes aegypti* mosquitoes. Am J Trop Med Hyg. 2005;72:616-621.

178. **Vicente T, Roldão A, Peixoto C,** et al. Large-scale production and purification of VLP- based vaccines. J Invertebr Pathol. 2011;107:42-8.

179. **Villatte F, Hussein AS, Bachmann TT,** et al. Expression level of heterologous proteins in *Pichia pastoris* is influenced by flask design. Appl Microbiol Biotechnol. 2001;55:463–465.

180. **Vogl T, Hartner FS, Glieder A.** New opportunities by synthetic biology for biopharmaceutical production in *Pichia pastoris*. Curr Opin Biotechnol. 2013;24:1094- 1101.

181. **Vrati S, Fernon CA, Dalgarno L,** et al. Location of a major antigenic site involved in ross river virus neutralization. Virology. 1988;162:346-53.

182. **Wang D, Suhrbier A, Penn-Nicholson A,** et al. A complex adenovirus vaccine against chikungunya virus provides complete protection against viraemia and arthritis. Vaccine. 2011; 9:2803-9.

183. **Wang E, Volkova E, Adams AP,** et al. Chimeric alphavirus vaccine candidates for chikungunya. Vaccine. 2008;26:5030-9.

184. **Weaver SC**. Vector Biology in Viral Pathogenesis. In: Nathanson, N., editor. Viral Pathogenesis. Lippincott-Raven; New York: 1997;329-352.

185. **Weaver SC and William KR**. Present and Future Arboviral Threats. Antiviral Res. 2010;85:328.

186. **Weaver SC, Osorio JE, Livengood JA,** et al. Chikungunya virus and prospects for a vaccine. Expert Rev Vaccines. 2012;11:1087-101.

187. **Werten MW, van den Bosch TJ, Wind RD,** et al. High-yield secretion of recombinant gelatins by *Pichia pastoris*. Yeast. 1999;15:1087–1096.

188. **Weiss B, Nitschko H, Ghattas I**, et al. Evidence for specificity in the encapsidation of Sindbis virus RNAs. J Virol. 1989;63:5310-8.

189. **Win MK, Chow A, Dimatatac F**, et al. Chikungunya fever in Singapore: Acute clinical laboratory features, and factors associated with persistent arthralgia. J Clin Virol. 2010;49:111–4.

190. Wu SR, Haag L, Sjöberg M, et al. The dynamic envelope of a fusion class II virus. E3 domain of glycoprotein E2 precursor in Semliki Forest virus provides a unique contact with the fusion protein E1. J Biol Chem. 2008;283**:**26452-60.

191. Xia M, Farkas T, Jiang X. Norovirus capsid protein expressed in yeast forms virus-like particles and stimulates systemic and mucosal immunity in mice following an oral administration of raw yeast extracts. J. Med. Virol 2007;79:74–83.

192. Yergolkar PN, Tandale BV, Arankalle VA, et al. Chikungunya outbreaks caused by African genotype, India. Emerg Infect Dis. 2006;12:1580-1583.

193. Zeller HG. Dengue, arbovirus and migrations in the Indian Ocean. Bull Soc Pathol Exot 1998;91:56-60.

194. Zhang R, Hryc CF, Cong Y, et al. 4.4 Å cryo-EM structure of an enveloped alphavirus Venezuelan equine encephalitis virus. EMBO J. 2011;30**:**3854-63.

APPENDICES

Reagents and Buffers

All reagents and buffers for nucleic acid and protein work were prepared in sterile Milli Q grade water. Cell culture media and reagents were sterilized by autoclaving for 15 min at 15-lb./sq. in. pressure unless otherwise mentioned.

Buffers for Agarose Gel Electrophoresis

- Tris Acetate EDTA (TAE) Buffer, pH 8.3 (50X) (per liter) Tris base 242 g

EDTA 18.6 g

Glacial acetic acid 57.1 ml

- Ethidium-bromide dye (10 mg/ml)

Reagents for SDS-PAGE

- Acrylamide (30 %)

Acrylamide 29.2 g

N, N' methylene bisacrylamide 0.8 g

Acrylamide was dissolved initially in 60 ml of Milli Q water and the volume was made up to 100 ml and the solution was filtered through Whattman filter paper no. 1 before use.

- Ammonium per sulfate 10% (w/v)
- TEMED 8.4% (v/v)
- Resolving buffer

Tris base 1M

Adjust pH to 8.8 with conc. HCl.

- Stacking buffer

Tris base 0.5M

Adjust pH to 6.8 with conc. HCl.

- Tris- Glycine buffer (per liter)

Tris base 3.03 g

Glycine 14.4g

SDS 1g

- Coomassie brilliant blue staining solution (per liter)

Brilliant blue (R250)	1 g	
Acetic acid		100 ml
Methanol		400 ml
Milli Q water		500 ml
(h) Destaining solution (per liter)		
Glacial acetic acid		100 ml
Methanol		400 ml
Milli Q water		500 ml

- **(i)** Lysis Buffer

Tris base 1.51 g

SDS 4 g

Glycine 20 g

Bromophenol blue 0.002 g

Dissolve in 60 ml of water and make up to 90 ml. Add 10 ml b-mercaptoethanol just before use.

Reagents for Western blot Analysis

(a) Transfer buffer (per liter)

Tris Base 3 g

Glycine 14.4 g

SDS 1g

Methanol 200 ml

(b) Blocking buffer 5% BSA in PBS

(c) Wash buffer 0.05% Tween 20 in PBS (PBS-T)

(d) Developing buffer

DAB 6 mg

1.1 M Citric acid 2.57 ml

1.2 M Na_2HPO_4 2.47 ml

MQ water 5 ml

30% H_2O_2 20 µl

Reagents for 96 well plate ELISA

- Coating buffer (pH 9.6)

Na_2CO_3 0.159 g

$NaHCO_3$ 0.290 g

Milli Q water 100 ml

- Blocking buffer 5% BSA in PBS
- Wash buffer 0.05% Tween 20 in PBS (PBS-T)

Buffers for Virus and VLPs Purification

(a)	GTNE buffer (pH 7.4)	
	Glycine	200nM
	NaCl	100mM
	Tris-HCl	50nM
	EDTA	1mM
(b)	20% Sucrose in GTNE buffer	
	Sucrose	20g
	GTNE buffer 80mL	
(c)	60% sucrose in GTNE buffer	
	Sucrose	60g
	GTNE buffer 50mL	

Media for Cell Culture

All standard media were prepared in milli Q water and sterilized by autoclaving for 20 min at 15 lbs/sq. in. pressure unless otherwise indicated.

(a) Eagles Minimum Essential Medium (EMEM) (per liter)

EMEM	9.4 g
$NaHCO_3$	2.0 g
Streptomycin	100 mg
Penicillin	100000 U
Gentamycin	40 mg
Milli Q water	900 ml

10 % Fetal bovine serum (FBS, Sigma) was added at the time of use to make complete EMEM.

(c) Overlay Medium Prepared in EMEM

Carboxymethyl cellulose	1.25%
FBS	2%
(d) Plaque Staining Solution Crystal violet	0.8%

Media for yeast culture

- YPD (Yeast extract Peptone dextrose) Media

Yeast extract	1%
Peptone	2%
Dextrose	2%

- Induction Media

Yeast extract	1%
Peptone	2%
Methanol	2%

INDEX

D

E

FSC
www.fsc.org
MIX
Papier | Fördert
gute Waldnutzung
FSC® C083411

Kolibri 360 GmbH
Ferdinand-Jühlke-Straße 7
99095 Erfurt, Deutschland
produktsicherheit@kolibri360.de